PRAISE FOR DELIVERING QU... ...
PEOPLE WITH DISABILITY

"The 61 million Americans with disability face significant health inequities and a healthcare workforce that is unprepared to meet their needs. Dr. Smeltzer has delivered a foundational, accessible, and practical text establishing that all healthcare providers have a role in—and need a basic understanding of—the issue of disability to provide appropriate, optimal, and sensitive healthcare to this marginalized population. This book is a must-read and an essential resource for all future nurses and healthcare providers at all levels."

–Susan M. Havercamp, PhD
Professor, Psychiatry and Behavioral Health
The Ohio State University Nisonger Center

"Suzanne Smeltzer has translated what she has learned in her life's work with people with disability into a thoughtful and comprehensive guide that can serve as a critical resource for nursing education programs and nurses in varied practice settings. Dr. Smeltzer masterfully synthesizes theory, research, and practice and provides clear strategies nurses can use to improve and humanize healthcare for people with disability."

–Alexa Stuifbergen, PhD, RN, FAAN
Dean, Laura Lee Blanton Chair
James Dougherty Jr. Centennial Professor in Nursing
The University of Texas at Austin School of Nursing

"This book is an essential read for healthcare providers of every discipline. How we choose to work with, learn from, and teach those with disability is a major challenge as we proclaim the need to overcome issues of diversity and inclusion in the year 2021. Dr. Smeltzer's work is in total alignment with the National League for Nursing's core values of caring, integrity, diversity and inclusion, and excellence."

–Beverly Malone, PhD, RN, FAAN
President and CEO, National League for Nursing

"Dr. Smeltzer's book, Delivering Quality Healthcare for People With Disability, *is a go-to resource for healthcare professionals. We fail to realize that those with disability comprise the largest minority group in the world, impacting 1 billion people globally. Smeltzer skillfully makes the argument why we need to do a better job in caring for those with disability and provides evidence-based information on a wide range of disabilities to assist us in achieving this goal."*

–Mary Ellen Smith Glasgow, PhD, RN, ACNS-BC, ANEF, FAAN
Dean and Professor, Duquesne University School of Nursing

"Dr. Smeltzer has been a pathfinder in delivering quality healthcare to people with disability. She has led national efforts to inform faculty in schools/colleges of nursing, both nationally and globally, to address the lack of knowledge, expertise, and experience to meet the unique needs of this vulnerable population. Her expertise is unparalleled, and this comprehensive and insightful book tackles a critical gap in the healthcare literature."

–M. Elaine Tagliareni, EdD, RN, CNE, FAAN
Dean and Professor, School of Nursing,
MGH Institute of Health Professions

"Dr. Smeltzer's book is a vital resource for the nursing profession as it strengthens its emphasis on population health. This crucial book along with her leadership in the field of disability nursing have enhanced nursing education's efforts to prepare knowledgeable and ethical practitioners to meet the health needs of people with disability. She also provides a blueprint for nursing practice to design and implement models of care that end health disparities for vulnerable populations."

–Dianne Cooney Miner, PhD, RN, FAAN
Dean Emeritus and Professor
Executive Director, Golisano Institute for Developmental Disabilities Nursing
St. John Fisher College

"A number of years ago, Dr. Smeltzer spoke at a national meeting after accepting an award for her pioneering work with individuals with disability. She gave life to the important work she was doing and opened my eyes to the unique challenges people with disability face. Her book, Delivering Healthcare for People With Disability, is clearly an important step in her journey to ensure that health providers and future providers understand best practices in caring for this population."

–Harriet R. Feldman, PhD, RN, FAAN
Dean and Professor
College of Health Professions and the Lienhard School of Nursing
Pace University

"Delivering Quality Healthcare for People With Disability, by Dr. Suzanne Smeltzer, with contributions from Dr. Beth Marks, is one of the first books to address this important health equity issue, which is unfortunately often overlooked in healthcare professional education. Key topics needing understanding by all healthcare professionals are addressed with practical advice on strategies for improvement."

–Sarah H. Ailey, PhD, RN, FAAN, PHNA-BC, CNE, CDDD
Professor, Rush University College of Nursing

DELIVERING QUALITY HEALTHCARE FOR PEOPLE WITH DISABILITY

SUZANNE C. SMELTZER, EdD, RN, ANEF, FAAN

Sigma
GLOBAL NURSING
EXCELLENCE

Sigma Theta Tau International Honor Society of Nursing (Sigma) is a nonprofit organization whose mission is developing nurse leaders anywhere to improve healthcare everywhere. Founded in 1922, Sigma has more than 135,000 active members in over 100 countries and territories. Members include practicing nurses, instructors, researchers, policymakers, entrepreneurs, and others. Sigma's more than 540 chapters are located at more than 700 institutions of higher education throughout Armenia, Australia, Botswana, Brazil, Canada, Colombia, Croatia, England, Eswatini, Ghana, Hong Kong, Ireland, Israel, Italy, Jamaica, Japan, Jordan, Kenya, Lebanon, Malawi, Mexico, the Netherlands, Nigeria, Pakistan, Philippines, Portugal, Puerto Rico, Scotland, Singapore, South Africa, South Korea, Sweden, Taiwan, Tanzania, Thailand, the United States, and Wales. Learn more at www.sigmanursing.org.

Sigma Theta Tau International
550 West North Street
Indianapolis, IN, USA 46202

To request a review copy for course adoption, order additional books, buy in bulk, or purchase for corporate use, contact Sigma Marketplace at 888.654.4968 (US/Canada toll-free), +1.317.687.2256 (International), or solutions@sigmamarketplace.org.

To request author information, or for speaker or other media requests, contact Sigma Marketing at 888.634.7575 (US/Canada toll-free) or +1.317.634.8171 (International).

ISBN: 9781948057455
EPUB ISBN: 9781948057462
PDF ISBN: 9781948057479
MOBI ISBN: 9781948057486

_____

Library of Congress Cataloging Number

LLCN
2020054398

_____

First Printing, 2021

Publisher: Dustin Sullivan   Managing Editor: Carla Hall
Acquisitions Editor: Emily Hatch   Project Editor: Kate Shoup
Development Editor: Kate Shoup   Copy Editor: Erin Geile
Cover Designer: Kim Scott, Bumpy Design   Proofreader: Gill Editorial Services
Interior Design/Page Layout: Rebecca Batchelor Indexer: Larry Sweazy

DEDICATION

This book is dedicated to those individuals with disability who have taught me more about life with a disability—and about life in general—than they will ever know or imagine. They have been wonderful, sharing teachers and have been the inspiration for this book. I hope it does justice to our shared goals of improving care to those with disability especially, but not limited to care provided by nurses.

ACKNOWLEDGMENTS

The author is grateful for the review of chapters of this book by the following nursing colleagues:

- Patricia K. Bradley, PhD, RN, FAAN, Villanova University M. Louise Fitzpatrick College of Nursing

- Jennifer Gunberg Ross, PhD, RN, CNE, Villanova University M. Louise Fitzpatrick College of Nursing

- Katherine Lucatorto, DNP, RN, Villanova University M. Louise Fitzpatrick College of Nursing

- Judith A. Stych, DNP, RN, CDDN, Nurse Consultant, Wisconsin Department of Health Services, Madison, WI

The author would also like to acknowledge the Villanova University's M. Louise Fitzpatrick College of Nursing "Team of Champions," who have adopted the goal of improved healthcare of individuals with disability through education of our nursing students to address this important issue.

ABOUT THE AUTHOR

SUZANNE C. SMELTZER, EdD, RN, ANEF, FAAN

Suzanne C. Smeltzer is the Richard and Marianne Kreider Endowed Professor in Nursing for Vulnerable Populations at Villanova University M. Louise Fitzpatrick College of Nursing. She has conducted research related to disability for more than 25 years and has presented multiple educational programs on the topic for healthcare professionals, professional organizations, and populations of individuals with disability She has served as a consultant to nursing faculty and schools of nursing on integration of disability in their curricula.

Smeltzer has received multiple awards for her work related to disability, including the 2016 Nurse.com/Gannett Foundation Lectureship Award for Diversity, Inclusion, and Sustainability in Nursing Education from the American Association of Colleges of Nursing. She was the first author/editor of *Brunner & Suddarth's Textbook of Medical-Surgical Nursing*, published by Lippincott Walters-Kluwer from 1992 to 2014, and continues to write the textbook's chapter on disability and chronic illness. This remains the only widely used medical-surgical nursing textbook that includes a section specifically on disability as well as disability-related issues throughout the book. The textbook has been translated into multiple languages and is used around the world. She was inducted into the American Academy of Nursing in 1992 and the Sigma International Nurse Researcher Hall of Fame in 2019 for her work on disability.

Smeltzer has been the driver of the standardized patients with disabilities project at Villanova University's College of Nursing, which ultimately resulted in the development of the Advancing Care Excellence for Persons with Disabilities (ACE.D) component of the National League for Nursing's series on advancing care excellence for vulnerable populations. She has had an active role in the development of competencies related to disability for nurses and other healthcare professionals. In addition, she has received research and programmatic funding related to disability and published widely on the issue. Her research has focused on attitudes of nurses toward individuals with disability, inclusion of disability-related content in nursing curricula and textbooks, and health issues of women with disability, including those related to pregnancy.

ABOUT THE CONTRIBUTING AUTHOR

BETH MARKS, PhD, RN, FAAN

Beth Marks, who contributed Chapter 9, is co-director of the HealthMatters Program, Associate Director for Research, Rehabilitation Research and Training Center on Aging with Developmental Disabilities (RRTCDD), and Research Associate Professor, Department of Disability and Human Development, College of Applied Health Sciences University of Illinois at Chicago.

Marks has addressed the lack of disability-related content and experiences in the education of most healthcare professionals and has had a prominent role in advocating for the inclusion of individuals with disability in nursing and nursing education. Many schools of nursing have automatically excluded from consideration applicants to their programs who disclose a disability. She views the inclusion of individuals with disability in nursing education and the retention of nurses with acquired disabilities in nursing practice as important strategies to increase nurses' understanding and knowledge about caring for individuals with disability they encounter in their practice. Marks's advice has been invaluable in working with faculty and administrators to determine what steps and strategies they should take to be fair to applicants and compliant with the law.

Marks coproduced *Open the Door, Get 'Em a Locker: Educating Nursing Students With Disabilities*, an award-winning documentary about the experiences of nursing students with disability. The documentary serves as a forum for voices of nursing students, faculty, academic administrators, and agency nursing staff to discuss the trials and triumphs of shifting perspectives and transforming nursing practice by healthcare providers with disability.

Marks has published and presented widely on the topic of disability and health professionals with disability, in journals and at conferences that reach multiple disciplines. She has been recognized for her contributions through a number of awards. She was inducted into the American Academy of Nursing for her contributions to nursing.

FREE RESOURCES

Visit the Sigma Repository for a two-page informational *Did you know* . . . flyer that contains quick facts and important reminders for all healthcare professionals providing direct or indirect care for people with disability.

Visit the page at http://hdl.handle.net/10755/20735 or simply scan the QR code below to go directly to the Repository page.

TABLE OF CONTENTS

1 DISABILITY: A MAJOR HEALTHCARE INEQUITY 1

2 THE ROLE OF SOCIAL DETERMINANTS OF HEALTH IN DISABILITY 19

3 STRATEGIES TO ADDRESS BARRIERS TO HEALTHCARE FOR PEOPLE WITH DISABILITY . . . 43

4 INTELLECTUAL AND DEVELOPMENTAL DISABILITIES 75

5 PHYSICAL DISABILITY 109

6 PSYCHIATRIC/MENTAL HEALTH DISABILITY AND NEUROCOGNITIVE DISORDERS 139

7 SENSORY DISABILITY: HEARING LOSS. 173

8 SENSORY DISABILITY: VISION LOSS 199

9 INCLUSION OF STUDENTS WITH DISABILITY: REDEFINING NURSING EDUCATION 229

INDEX 271

FOREWORD

Delivering Quality Healthcare for People With Disability, by Suzanne Smeltzer, with contributing author Beth Marks, is a must-read for nurse educators, advanced practice nurses, and students of the profession. Schools of nursing and medicine have not engaged in meaningful education about care of people with disability, and few schools of nursing or their graduate programs adequately address the health and healthcare issues of individuals with disability. At the undergraduate level, care of people with disability may be discussed in courses that address infants, children, and adults with genetic illnesses. In the care of the adult or in geriatric nursing, students learn about movement disorders associated with neurological or cardiovascular diseases and the impact of traumatic injuries such as motor vehicle crashes, falls, and gunshot wounds on mobility and cognition. Some schools offer simulations programs in which students are "given" disabilities and asked to navigate their environment with blindfolds, padded earphones, crutches, or with one arm in a sling, a practice discouraged by the disability community and disability advocates.

Although nursing students care for people with disability, the focus of care is usually on the management of acute or chronic illness and the provision of safety or comfort measures. Few nursing course objectives emphasize the Alliance for Disability in Health Care Education's Core Competencies on Disability for Health Care Education (2019). Course readings seldom mention global and national reports on the scope of disabilities by the World Health Organization, the International Council of Nurses, or the National Academy of Medicine. Few nursing education programs address the interaction of disability and healthcare or the barriers to quality healthcare experienced by individuals with disability.

This book covers disability as an inequity and a health disparity within the context of social determinants of health, noting that disability can be intellectual, developmental, or physical, as well as expressions of neurological disorders, mental illnesses, or sensory impairments. One significant chapter of the book speaks to the fact that nursing students can also be living with disabilities.

Globally, more than a billion people, about 15% of the world's population, live with some form of disability (World Health Organization, 2018). In the United States, one in four persons have a disability (Centers for Disease Control and Prevention, 2018). Yet definitions, classifications, and the epidemiology of disability do not receive adequate attention in nursing education and practice. Dr. Smeltzer not only identifies this problem but also provides strategies to bring about curriculum change. Given the number of people with disability, the gaps in nursing education must be addressed.

People with disability are the largest group of vulnerable persons in the United States. Most Americans have or know someone with a disability. Dr. Smeltzer gives a face to the statistics by describing how disabilities are commonly associated with mobility, cognition, hearing, vision, and the ability to live alone or engage in self-care.

The book also charts how the US has changed its approach to people with disability. Some live with their parents or relatives. Others live in group homes with other adults with mobility issues or cognitive difficulties. In the past, some people with disability were placed in institutions—often long-term psychiatric hospitals. Some became homeless or found themselves in jail.

Today most young people with disability are successfully mainstreamed in primary and secondary schools. Students assisted by mobility devices and students who rely on interpreters to help them understand what their teachers and classmates are saying graduate higher education. Despite these successes, healthcare for those with disability often remains problematic and inadequate.

This book is more than a textbook. It is a road map to overcoming a noticeable gap in the education of health professionals. It increases awareness and deepens the knowledge base of professional nurses and students. Knowledge and physical barriers can be improved, and

I encourage you to read and have your students and colleagues read *Delivering Quality Healthcare for People With Disability.*

–Sr. Rosemary Donley, PhD, APRN, FAAN
Professor of Nursing and the Jacques Laval Chair for
Justice for Vulnerable Populations
Duquesne University

REFERENCES

Alliance for Disability in Health Care Education. (2019). *Core Competencies on Disability for Health Care Education.* Retrieved from http://www.adhce.org/resources/core-competencies-on-disability-for-health-care-education/

Centers for Disease Control and Prevention. (2018). *Disability impacts all of us.* Retrieved from https://www.cdc.gov/ncbddd/disabilityandhealth/infographic-disability-impacts-all.html#:~:text=61%20million%20adults%20in%20the,have%20some%20type%20of%20disability

World Health Organization. (2018). *Disability and health.* Retrieved from https://www.who.int/news-room/fact-sheets/detail/disability-and-health

INTRODUCTION

"Disability is a universal aspect of human experience, affecting nearly everyone at some point in his or her life span."

–Kirschner & Curry, 2009

In 2009, in a commentary published in the *Journal of the American Medical Association,* Kirschner and Curry stated what should be obvious to all of us: Disability is a universal aspect of human experience, and it will affect all of us, either directly or indirectly, at some point in our lives. Despite its universality and the inevitable encounters with disability that nurses and other healthcare professionals will have—personally and as part of their role as health professionals—the health professions' educational programs do not adequately prepare students to provide quality care to individuals with disability.

Those with disability—be it mild and a mere inconvenience, or one that necessitates the use of high-tech support for survival—have repeatedly reported that their healthcare needs are not adequately addressed by healthcare providers. Most healthcare professionals, including nurses, are unfamiliar with the consequences of disabling conditions in the lives of individuals with disability. They lack knowledge about how to communicate effectively with those with all types of disability, do not consider the effect of individuals' disability on their ability to participate in health-promotion efforts, harbor negative attitudes and bias toward them, stereotype them, and often perceive them as unable (or unwilling) to take an active part in their own care.

Healthcare professionals have reported that disability is not a very important issue, despite the statistics that indicate that people with disability comprise the largest minority group in the US. Some healthcare providers have indicated that they are unlikely to be in roles or settings in which they will care for individuals with disability, when in fact, based on the large and growing number of people with disability and their need and desire for healthcare, they are very likely to encounter individuals with disability in their practice.

Many healthcare professionals recognize and acknowledge that they lack knowledge, expertise, and experience to provide quality care for this population, despite years of education to prepare them to provide quality healthcare to diverse populations. Because of this lack of knowledge and expertise on the part of healthcare professionals across healthcare settings, communication and interaction of healthcare providers with individuals with disability, and the healthcare they receive, remain very problematic.

Ineffective communication on the part of healthcare professionals when interacting with individuals with disability has broad implications and repercussions. Healthcare providers who believe they know best, and are the experts on disability (despite their acknowledged lack of expertise on the topic), will continue to ignore the wishes and preferences of individuals with disability and their desire to make decisions about their own lives and healthcare. Many healthcare professionals presume people with disability are reluctant to participate in health promotion. Many healthcare professionals are unaware of barriers to accessible healthcare and screening experienced by individuals with disability, and as a result are unable to identify ways to address or overcome those barriers. Healthcare professionals who do not understand disability and the contributions that those with disability make to their families, to the lives of others, and to society as a whole, may consider preventive health screening and health promotion efforts to be not worth the effort for someone who already has a disability.

Individuals with disability have reported that healthcare providers are uncomfortable and unwilling to discuss issues related to sex and sexuality with them. They have further reported that healthcare providers assume that they are uninterested (or perhaps believe that they should be uninterested) in sexual relationships, intimacy, pregnancy, and childbearing. Women with disability who have elected to become mothers and have sought out prenatal care have reported that their healthcare providers' first assumption was that the reason for their healthcare visit was to terminate their pregnancy, even if the pregnancy was well-thought-out and planned. Women with disability who have successfully become pregnant have been questioned and chastised by healthcare professionals about their decision to bear children, and have even been blatantly accused of being irresponsible for becoming pregnant and having children. Women with disability have expressed fear that someone will attempt to remove their children from them based solely on their having a disability, regardless of how well they have cared for their children and been very successful and effective parents.

Most studies that have addressed the healthcare experiences of individuals with disability have focused on their interactions with physicians. However, studies of nurses indicate that nurses' attitudes and knowledge level mirror those of physicians and reflect those of greater society. Numerous national and global organizations and agencies have issued calls for the healthcare disciplines to address the inadequate healthcare experienced by individuals with disability; these agencies and organizations have identified changing the educational preparation of healthcare professionals as a primary strategy and an important first step.

Several organizations, with input from individuals with disability, have developed competencies that should be expected of all healthcare professionals who interact with individuals with disability. The Alliance for Disability in Health Care Education has urged nursing, medicine, and other healthcare professions to endorse these competencies with the goal of moving forward in the effort to improve the healthcare of individuals with disability. Nurses have been very involved in the development of these competencies from the beginning of the process. Several nursing

Throughout this book, the authors use the term *people with disability* rather than *people with disabilities*. The singular disability is used as a collective noun to note commonalities rather than differences among individuals with different types of disability or groups of individuals with disability. The term disabilities has been avoided because it suggests differences and fragmentation rather than the similarities that this book is intended to address (McDermott & Turk, 2014).

organizations, including Sigma, have endorsed the cross-discipline competencies developed by the Alliance for Disability in Health Care Education (2019).

This book is based on the principle and belief that all healthcare professionals—regardless of discipline, level of education, or role within the healthcare system—have a role in caring for individuals with disability. As such, they need a basic understanding of the issue of disability to provide appropriate, optimal, and sensitive healthcare to those with disability. These issues and more are addressed in the chapters of this book. It is intended to provide information to nurses, nursing students, and other healthcare professionals to enable them to communicate with and provide quality healthcare to individuals with disability.

The first three chapters of this book provide essential background information intended to put the topic of disability in context. Often, disability is not the reason that an individual with a disability seeks healthcare. However, the presence of a disability often has a negative effect on the individual's interaction with healthcare clinicians. The goal of this book's first three chapters is to provide background to ensure that interactions with those with disability are positive and of high quality. The first three chapters also provide definitions of important terms and an explanation of what terms are considered acceptable by individuals with disability and their community.

Key information addressed in Chapter 1 includes the epidemiology of disability and an explanation of the major categories of disability. This illustrates that types of disability have been categorized in many ways over time, and some terms have been discarded as objectionable.

Chapter 2 discusses the social determinants of health. These can have a very significant impact on how individuals with disability are perceived and are treated within the healthcare system. A historical view of models of disability and the role of these models in framing the views of healthcare professionals and the broader society are also discussed. In addition, an important distinction is made between "disability" and "disabling condition." Nurses and other healthcare professionals can be very knowledgeable about a disabling condition without considering the day-to-day experience of individuals with disability as they try to navigate a healthcare system that frequently throws barriers in their way to obtaining care. To put today's approaches to disability in historical perspective, a brief history of disability through the ages is included. Finally, strategies for communicating with individuals with various types of disability are discussed.

Chapter 3 introduces barriers to access to healthcare for individuals with disability. These have been identified by multiple agencies, researchers, and individuals with disability and their advocates. Specific categories of barriers are addressed, along with the consequences of those barriers on access to healthcare. Strategies to address these barriers are suggested. Important federal legislation related to the rights of individuals with disability is also addressed.

Each of the next five chapters discusses a major category of disability. This is to provide nursing students and nurses in practice with the necessary background to communicate with and care for individuals with that disability. Each chapter provides information about the disability category; appropriate terminology; and information about the prevalence, causes, and consequences of disabilities in that category. They also provide examples of specific disabling conditions within the category of disability, along with specific points about caring for individuals with disabilities in that category. Finally, each chapter includes links to informative and helpful resources. It is not the author's intention to make readers experts or specialists in disability. Rather, it is to arm them with information that will enable them to provide high-quality and sensitive care to individuals with disability they see in their practice across various settings. These include but are not limited to outpatient settings, acute and long-term care facilities, maternity settings, and home- and community-based settings.

The last chapter of the book, Chapter 9, addresses the inclusion of individuals with disability in nursing education. The discussion is based in part on the principle that nursing care—and, more generally, healthcare—could be improved and made more accessible, more welcoming, and more effective for individuals with disability if healthcare providers knew about disability from their own personal experience and perspective. Hopefully, the information included in this chapter will result in more open, welcoming, and supportive admission policies to enable individuals with disability to become nurses and other healthcare professionals and to improve the health and nursing care of this population in the future.

This book is based on the principle and belief that all healthcare providers have a role in caring for people with disability and need a basic understanding of the issue of disability to provide appropriate, optimal, and sensitive healthcare to those with disability. The hope is that this book will serve as a starting point for nursing students, nurses in practice, nursing faculty, and others interested in the topic of disability to consider the healthcare issues experienced by individuals with disability, at least in part because of barriers to quality care. I want the nursing discipline in general and nurses in particular to take the lead in addressing the needs of people with disability in our care. Nursing and nurses must become the solution, rather than part of the problem, for individuals with disability seeking healthcare.

COVID-19 AND PEOPLE WITH DISABILITY

This book was written in part during the worldwide coronavirus (Covid-19) pandemic that surged in 2020. The pandemic raised important issues for individuals with disability, their families, and other support persons, as well as for nurses and other healthcare providers who provide healthcare to all populations. The Covid-19 pandemic has affected individuals with disability more than many other populations.

In the best of circumstances—that is, in the absence of a pandemic like Covid-19—people with disability experience healthcare inequities. They have a difficult time obtaining the kind of healthcare they need and deserve. Some healthcare providers fail to recognize the desire and ability of individuals with disability to have a say in what happens to them when they seek healthcare and do not treat individuals with disability with the dignity and respect they deserve. Although the Americans with Disabilities Act was passed more than 30 years ago, in 1990, many changes and policies are still needed to ensure that healthcare for this population is available, accessible, respectful, and sensitive to their needs.

The Covid-19 pandemic uncovered even more issues that need to be addressed. One of these is that in many cases, people with disability are at increased risk for Covid-19 infection because of preexisting health conditions—often multiple health conditions. Some of these preexisting conditions put people with disability at high risk in ordinary circumstances because many have what could be considered a narrow margin of safety or health. Although disability cannot and should not be equated with poor health, this narrow margin of safety may make it more likely that someone with disability will experience health issues earlier or more easily than others. For example, if someone has a high spinal cord injury, that person's respiratory status may be good in normal circumstances, enabling him or her to breathe without difficulty. But if that individual has a simple respiratory infection (or cold), his or her respiratory status may become compromised more easily. Then, when the severe respiratory symptoms that often occur with Covid-19 develop, the likelihood of severe respiratory failure increases dramatically.

The Covid-19 pandemic has created other problems for people with disability. For example, during the pandemic, people with disability have been justifiably concerned that they might not be seen as deserving of hospitalization and ICU care, including treatment with ventilators, if needed. The pandemic has also made it increasingly more difficult for individuals with disability to obtain other treatments they might need, as well as food, medication, and other products required to maintain their well-being.

The ability of individuals with mobility limitations to wash their hands may be reduced. Although hand sanitizers can be used in these situations, the limited supply or availability of such sanitizers may prevent individuals with disability from using them as often as recommended. Further, handwashing with soap and water is preferable and more effective than using hand sanitizers.

During the Covid-19 pandemic, some healthcare facilities established policies prohibiting family members or other support persons from staying with patients during hospitalization in an effort to decrease the risk of virus transmission. This was devastating for many individuals who required hospitalization, including those with disability—particularly for those with intellectual or cognitive disability and those who have difficulty communicating with healthcare team members. These individuals often require additional time to communicate and frequently rely on family members or support persons to assist them. Family members or support persons are also often needed to minimize the stress and anxiety that arises in hectic or chaotic situations, such as acute care or emergency room visits.

The pandemic has also affected people with hearing loss because of the need for healthcare providers—and everyone else—to wear masks. Masks prevent people with hearing loss who rely on facial expressions and lip/speech reading from understanding what others are saying. When wearing a mask, healthcare providers must use new strategies to communicate with people with hearing loss.

The effects of Covid-19 in nursing homes and other long-term care facilities during the pandemic have been tragic and distressing. The pandemic has placed individuals with disability who live in nursing homes or long-term facilities at increased risk due to their close proximity with others and an inability to maintain social distancing. Employees in nursing homes and other long-term care facilities—which are often understaffed—are also at increased risk for infection. This is due to their own health issues, a lack of personal resources, the fact that many of them are underserved in their own communities, a lack of personal protective equipment (PPE), and the frequency with which they provide close physical care to residents. Moreover, many staff members use public transportation to get to their jobs, increasing their exposure to people who may be infected. All these factors contribute to the risk of transmission of Covid-19 to both residents and caregivers, resulting in the tragic events that have occurred in nursing homes and long-term care facilities nationwide.

The lack of preparation for the Covid-19 pandemic in 2020 has taken many people and organizations by surprise. Going forward, analyses of what went wrong and what can be done to prevent the recurrence of the devastation experienced in nursing homes and long-term care facilities, and by society as a whole, are crucial. As a country and as healthcare professionals, we must recognize that pandemics are possible and prepare for them accordingly. We must also ensure that organizations such as the Centers for Disease Control and Prevention and healthcare departments across the country have the resources they need to conduct appropriate surveillance and to develop evidence-based policies needed to contain pandemics. Simply put, we must have a coordinated response within healthcare and across the country.

REFERENCES

Alliance for Disability in Health Care Education. (2019). Core competencies on disability for health care education. Retrieved from https://nisonger.osu.edu/wp-content/uploads/2019/08/post-consensus-Core-Competencies-on-Disability_8.5.19.pdf

Kirschner, K. L., & Curry, R. H. (2009). Educating health care professionals to care for patients with disabilities. *Journal of the American Medical Association, 302*(12), 1,334–1,335. doi:10.1001/jama.2009.1398

McDermott, S., & Turk, M. A. (2014). Disability language in the Disability and Health Journal. *Disability and Health Journal, 7*(3), 257–258. doi:10.1016/j.dhjo.2014.05.002

1
DISABILITY: A MAJOR HEALTHCARE INEQUITY

INTRODUCTION

Disability affects more than 1 billion people globally. These include more than 61 million people living in the United States. This translates to one in every four noninstitutionalized residents of the US (Okoro, Hollis, Cyrus, & Griffin-Blake, 2018; Office of the Surgeon General & Office on Disability, 2005; World Health Organization [WHO], 2011). The prevalence of disability continues to increase over time (Iezzoni, Kurtz, & Rao, 2014; Okoro et al., 2018). Still, these statistics likely underestimate the number of people with disability because they do not include those who live in institutions or are active duty military personnel. Based on these statistics, the population of people with disability is the largest minority group (United Nations, 2019).

Disability occurs in every age group across the life span, in every community, in every racial and ethnic group, and in every socioeconomic category. Disability can be visible or invisible (or not apparent to others). It can range from mild, with little effect on function, to very severe, necessitating support for survival. This includes support from others as well as technological support.

Multiple studies have reported that people with disability across all these groups receive healthcare that is inferior to that received by those without disability. People with disability encounter multiple barriers to optimal health and quality healthcare. They are more likely than people without disability to report lack of access to healthcare, less participation in preventive health screening (including Pap tests, mammograms, and bone density tests), less involvement in health promotion activities, and greater susceptibility to preventable health problems. All these can lead to overall poor health and poor quality of life.

The social determinants of health contribute to the inequities in health and healthcare experienced by people with disability. See Chapter 2 for further discussion of this issue.

THE NEED FOR IMPROVED HEALTHCARE FOR PEOPLE WITH DISABILITY

Disability and the health-related needs of people with disability are not adequately addressed by the healthcare disciplines, including nursing. This important topic must be addressed by all healthcare professions, including nursing and nursing education, to prepare future generations of health professionals to provide quality healthcare to those with disability. The high prevalence of disability across the globe and in the US is reason enough to justify greater attention to disability in nursing, from nursing education to practice to administration and research.

Because the topic of disability is not well addressed by any group or category of health professionals, the nursing profession has the opportunity to take the lead in addressing disability in the education and training of future nurses and other healthcare professionals, in participating in interprofessional care and collaboration with colleagues from other disciplines, in changing institutional policies, and in advocating for policy change to improve the healthcare and healthcare access of people with disability.

Multiple calls to action have been issued urging healthcare professionals to improve the inadequate healthcare provided to people with disability. (See the following sidebar.) One major strategy strongly recommended in these calls to action is to improve the education and training of health professionals so they are prepared to provide high-quality, sensitive care to those with disability. Despite these calls and their urgency, the healthcare professions as a whole have been slow to take steps to address disability in their education and training programs. This book is designed to provide healthcare professionals—including nursing students, clinicians, and faculty—with information needed to provide quality care to people with disability.

CALLS TO ACTION TO IMPROVE HEALTHCARE FOR PEOPLE WITH DISABILITY

- Office of the Surgeon General Reports (2002, 2005)
- Institute of Medicine (IOM) Report on Disability (2007)
- National Council on Disability Report (2009)
- World Health Organization (WHO) World Report on Disability (2011)
- International Council of Nurses (ICN) Position Paper (2000, 2010)
- Patient Protection and Affordable Care Act (2010)
- UN Flagship Report on Disability and Development (United Nations, 2018)

In addition to these calls for action, the General Assembly of the United Nations adopted an important resolution addressing the rights of people with disability around the world. The Convention on the Rights of Persons with Disabilities (CRPD), GA resolution A/RES/61/106 (United Nations, 2006), is an international human rights treaty that was adopted in 2006, opened for endorsement by countries around the world in 2007, and enacted in 2008. Specific articles of the CRPD call for access to equitable healthcare for people with disability. Although the resolution is considered a major step forward in the elimination of discrimination against people with disability around the world, including in access to healthcare, many countries, including the United States, have yet to sign onto the resolution.

Healthcare providers in every setting—from outpatient clinics, to home and community settings, to hospitals and intensive care settings—will encounter people with disability and must be prepared to provide high-quality healthcare for them. Although some health-care professionals are more likely to see people with disability in their clinical practice than others, knowledge and skill in providing healthcare for those with disability should be part of *every* health-care providers' education and training (Kirschner & Curry, 2009).

Knowledge about disability should be considered a responsibility of all providers—not only those with a special interest in disability.

This book is based on the principle and belief that all healthcare providers have a role in caring for people with disability and need a basic understanding of the issue of disability to provide appropriate, optimal, and sensitive healthcare to those with disability. These issues and more are addressed in this chapter and those that follow. In addition, disability is discussed as it relates to nursing students and nursing school applicants with disability.

DEFINING DISABILITY

Before identifying strategies to improve healthcare for this population, it is important first to define what is meant by disability. Although many definitions of disability exist, there is consensus that disability is neither a health problem alone nor an illness. Rather, *disability* is generally viewed as the effect of physical, mental, sensory, or cognitive/intellectual impairment on one's general well-being and on one's ability to participate in activities that other people can easily do (combined with environmental factors that hinder that participation).

An important definition of disability is that of the World Health Organization (WHO), which developed the International Classification of Functioning, Disability and Health (ICF) to define and characterize disability (WHO, 2001). With the development of the ICF, the WHO moved away from its previous focus on disease to a focus on health. This new focus addresses factors that affect the day-to-day life of a person with a disability, with the goal of identifying and addressing those factors.

The WHO ICF definition of disability addresses components of health and physical and mental well-being, as well as education and employment.

The ICF identifies *disability* as an umbrella term for impairments to functioning, activity limitations, or participation restrictions, where (WHO, 2011):

- *Impairment* is a problem in body function or structure.

- *Functioning* refers to all body functions, activities, and participation.

- *Activity limitation* is a difficulty or barrier that affects a person's ability to carry out a task or an action.

- *Participation restriction* describes a factor or issue that affects one's ability to be involved in usual life situations and activities.

The ICF also addresses environmental factors that interact with these factors. So, in simple terms, the focus of the WHO definition of disability, then, is on the *interaction* of a person with a health condition and the personal and environmental factors that affect the person's day-to-day life and well-being. To be more specific, the WHO defines *disability* as the interaction between people with disabling conditions—such as cerebral palsy, spinal cord injury, or autism spectrum disorder—and factors that affect their ability to carry out activities of daily living (ADLs) and to obtain appropriate healthcare. These factors could include (but are not limited to):

- Negative attitudes on the part of healthcare providers about people with disability

- Healthcare providers' lack of knowledge about disability

- Inaccessible or unreliable transportation

- Healthcare facilities or clinicians' offices that are not barrier-free

- Limited social supports and services

Although the WHO definition might seem cumbersome at first, it is designed to focus on factors that can be modified to improve access of people with disability to the same activities that are available to others: healthcare, education, work, and family and community activities.

Like the WHO, the International Council of Nurses (ICN) has also issued a definition of disability and described nurses' role in caring for people with disability. This was put forth in a position statement in 2000, which was reviewed and revised in 2010. The ICN defines disability as a physical, mental, sensory, or social impairment that, in the long term, adversely affects one's ability to carry out normal day-to-day activities (ICN, 2000, 2010). The ICN's position statement also identifies the important role of nurses in caring for people with disability. The discussion of nurses' role in caring for individuals with disability reflects the positions of the ICN.

In the United States, we often use the definition of disability from the Americans with Disabilities Act (ADA) of 1990. This definition is one that nurses and other healthcare professionals should know because it has legal implications. The ADA defines *disability* as a physical or mental impairment that substantially limits one or more major life activities, a record or history of such an impairment, *or* a case in which someone is regarded or viewed by others as having such an impairment (Americans with Disabilities Act, 1990). The ADA and other legislation and policy that are relevant to disability will be discussed in subsequent chapters of this book.

Different definitions of disability are needed and used for different purposes for healthcare, education, and employment. For example, specific definitions and criteria are needed in educational settings to determine whether the presence or severity of a disability qualifies a student for supports and services to ensure optimal learning and functioning in the school environment. Other definitions of disability are needed to determine if a person qualifies for financial and other support through an employer, for federal support for healthcare through Medicare (Centers for Medicare and Medicaid Services, 2019), for health insurance coverage, or for disability services through the Social Security Administration.

Table 1.1 presents these and other important definitions of disability.

TABLE 1.1   DEFINITIONS OF DISABILITY

SOURCE	DEFINITION
Americans with Disabilities Act (1990)	A physical or mental impairment that substantially limits one or more major life activities, a record or history of such an impairment, or a case in which someone is regarded or viewed by others as having such an impairment
International Council of Nurses (2010)	A physical, mental, sensory, or social impairment that, in the long term, adversely affects one's ability to carry out normal day-to-day activities
Social Security Administration (SSA) (2020)	A severe impairment that has either lasted or can be expected to last for a minimum of one year An impairment severe enough to prevent a person from engaging in substantial and gainful activity (SGA). SGA is a term used by the SSA to describe a level of work activity and earnings. *Substantial* refers to significant physical or mental activities or a combination of both (could be full- or part-time); *gainful* refers to work performed for pay or profit.
US Department of Education Individuals with Disabilities Education Act (2018)	The Individuals with Disabilities Education Act (IDEA) considers a child to have a disability if that child has an intellectual disability, a hearing impairment, a speech or language impairment, a visual impairment, a serious emotional disturbance, an orthopedic impairment, autism spectrum disorder, traumatic brain injury, another health impairment, a specific learning disability, deaf-blindness, or multiple disabilities, who requires special education and related services.
World Health Organization/ICF (2011)	An umbrella term for impairments to functioning, activity limitations, and participation restrictions; includes environmental factors that interact with all these components

TYPES OF DISABILITIES

There are many different categories of disability and many different specific disabilities and disabling conditions. (Chapter 2 discusses the difference between the terms *disability* and *disabling condition.*)

One way to categorize disability is by age of onset—in other words, during and after the developmental years. These categories are as follows:

- **Developmental disabilities:** These occur during a person's developmental years—that is, before 22 years of age (National Institutes of Health, 2010). A *developmental disability* is a severe, long-term disability that can affect cognitive ability, physical functioning, or both. Some developmental disabilities involve only physical impairments, such as osteogenesis imperfecta or blindness. Other developmental disabilities can result in both physical and intellectual impairments, such as cerebral palsy and Down syndrome. Developmental disabilities that affect cognitive function are identified as intellectual disabilities (American Association on Intellectual and Developmental Disabilities [AAIDD], 2012). Some developmental disabilities are present at or before birth and may be due to genetic factors; these are also referred to as *congenital disabilities* or anomalies (WHO, 2016). Spina bifida, for example, is a congenital disorder that occurs when the spinal column does not form properly during fetal development, leaving the spinal cord and spinal nerves exposed through an opening along the spinal column (National Institute of Neurological Disorders and Stroke, 2019).

- **Intellectual disabilities:** These are developmental disabilities characterized by impaired cognitive (or intellectual) function and difficulty with adaptive behaviors or activities such as managing money, maintaining schedules and routines, and engaging in interactions with others. These disabilities originate before the age of 18 and may or may not be associated with physical impairment. Fragile X syndrome, Down syndrome, and autism spectrum disorder are examples of disabilities that affect a person's cognitive function and adaptive behaviors (AAIDD, 2012).

- **Acquired disabilities:** These are disabilities that arise at any time after the developmental years—that is, after 22 years of age. Examples of acquired disabilities are impairments resulting from such conditions as multiple sclerosis, spinal cord injury, stroke, severe obstructive lung disease, Alzheimer's disease and other dementias, or amputation due to a traumatic injury or chronic disease such as diabetes.

Another way of categorizing disability is by the major function that is affected. Using this method, functional types of disability may be categorized as mobility, cognitive, independent living, vision, hearing, and self-care (Courtney-Long et al., 2015).

A single disability can be categorized several ways and may fit several definitions of disability. For example, a stroke, which is an acquired disability, can result in physical or mobility disability, cognitive disability, and communication/speech and language disability. Another example is sensory disability. *Sensory disabilities* impair the senses (i.e., vision, hearing, smell, taste, and touch). Because 95% of the information we receive is through sight and hearing, impairments of these senses can have a great impact on learning and communication. Sensory disabilities are considered developmental disabilities if they arise before 22 years of age. If they arise after 22 years of age or in aging adults, they are considered acquired disabilities.

IMPORTANT TERMINOLOGY

There are numerous other categories of disabilities and additional terms that healthcare professionals need to be familiar with to understand disability and its impact on those affected and their families. Table 1.2 presents important terms, including the major types of disability. It is important to note that there is overlap among these terms. The major categories and examples of disabilities will be discussed in subsequent chapters of this book.

TABLE 1.2   DISABILITY-RELATED TERMS AND TYPES OF DISABILITY

TERM	DESCRIPTION
Acquired disability	Impairment that occurs at any time after the developmental years; may be due to injury or disease; examples are spinal cord injury, multiple sclerosis, stroke, and amputation due to trauma or complications of diabetes
Cognitive impairment (CDC, 2011)	An impairment in the ability to remember, learn new things, concentrate, or make decisions that affect everyday life; may be mild or severe; may occur with Alzheimer's disease or other dementias or traumatic brain injury
Communication/speech and language disability (CDC, n.d.-d; NIH, 2019)	Impaired ability to receive, send, process, and comprehend concepts or verbal, nonverbal, or graphic symbol systems; may be primary disability or secondary to other disabilities May be a speech disorder (an impairment of the articulation of speech sounds, fluency or voice) or a language disorder (impaired comprehension and use of spoken, written, or other symbol systems)
Congenital disability	Impairment present at or before birth; can occur during the fetal stage of development, from injury or infection that occurs during pregnancy or from genetic factors; a type of developmental disability
Developmental disability (CDC, n.d.-a; National Institutes of Health, 2010)	Impairment in physical, learning, language, or behavior areas that begins during the developmental period (up to 22 years of age); may affect day-to-day functioning; usually lasts throughout a person's lifetime; can involve intellectual disability alone, physical or sensory disability alone, or both physical and intellectual disabilities
Functioning (WHO/ICF)	An umbrella term encompassing all body functions, activities, and participation
Hearing impairment, hearing loss, or deafness (CDC, n.d.-e)	Impairment in hearing or hearing loss; severity is based on loss of ability to hear levels of sound measured in decibels Individuals who develop hearing loss later in life are referred to as having hearing impairment or are deaf, depending on extent of hearing loss

continues

TABLE 1.2   DISABILITY-RELATED TERMS AND TYPES OF DISABILITY (CONT.)

TERM	DESCRIPTION
Impairment (WHO/ICF)	A problem in body function or structure
Intellectual disability (CDC, n.d.-b; NIH, 2010)	Impairment of mental capacity and often difficulty with adaptive behaviors such as managing money, schedules and routines, or social interactions; occurs before the age of 18; intellectual disability is one example of developmental disability The term *learning disability* is used in some countries instead of intellectual disability.
International Classification of Functioning, Disability and Health (WHO/ICF)	A classification of health and health-related domains that helps describe changes in body function and structure, what people with a health condition can do in a standard environment (their level of capacity), as well as what they actually do in their usual environment (their level of performance)
Limitation, activity (WHO/ICF)	A difficulty or barrier that affects a person's ability to carry out a task or an action
Participation restriction (WHO/ICF)	A factor or issue that affects one's ability to be involved in usual life situations
Physical or motor disability	Impairment that affects one's ability to carry out physical activities, including mobility; may require assistance from others or use of assistive devices; may result from birth defects, disease, aging, or injury
Psychiatric disability (ADA, 1990)	A mental impairment or illness that significantly interferes with being able to complete major life activities, such as learning, working, and communicating
Sensory disability	Impairment of the senses (i.e., sight, hearing, smell, touch, or taste); most commonly refers to impairment of vision or hearing
Vision impairment, vision loss, or blindness (CDC, n.d.-d)	Impairment in vision; can be mild and correctable or severe and not correctable to a "normal" level

EPIDEMIOLOGY OF DISABILITY

In the past, it has been difficult even to estimate the number of people with disability because they were often missed in data collection efforts used to determine prevalence rates. In addition, the presence of a disability has often been an exclusion criterion in studies. However, it is believed that more than 1 billion people live with a disability—approximately 15% of the world's population. Of these, 95 million are children between 0 and 14 years of age, or 5.1% of the global population of children (Institute for Health Metrics and Evaluation, 2019), with 13 million having severe disability. More than 975 million people 15 years of age and older worldwide live with one or more disabilities, including 110 to 190 million people with severe disability. These figures represent an increasing prevalence of disability around the world, due in part to the aging population and increases in chronic health conditions, including obesity (WHO, 2018).

> Although one person in a family may have a disability, the disability likely affects all members of a family and perhaps the community in a variety of ways.

The prevalence of disability varies by country, regions within countries, age, racial/ethnic groups, gender, socioeconomic status, and sexual orientation. The percentage of children (< 18 years of age) in the US with disability is 17.1%, with 9.8% having severe disability. The prevalence of severe disability and the need for personal assistance increase with age. Although the probability of having a severe disability is less than 1 in 10 adults between 18 and 24 years of age, the number increases to 3 in 10 for adults between 60 and 65 years of age. Almost 54% of adults 75 years of age and older have a severe disability (Courtney-Long et al., 2015). Black, non-Hispanic adults reported the highest prevalence of disability and of each disability type in the US. Disability is more common in the southern states of the US and in adults with lower incomes and adults who did not complete high school. Lesbian, gay, and bisexual older adults have higher rates of disability, as do older adults living in rural settings. Table 1.3 outlines the prevalence of disability in the US and includes a breakdown by age, race, and gender.

TABLE 1.3 PREVALENCE OF DISABILITY IN THE US (TOTAL AND BY AGE, RACE, AND GENDER)

TOTAL PREVALENCE OF DISABILITY	PERCENT
Total US population	27.2
DISABILITIES BY AGE GROUP	**PERCENT**
< 18 years of age	17.1
18–64 years of age	23.7
65–74 years or age	58.5
≥ 75 years and older	70.5
DISABILITIES BY RACE	**PERCENT**
White, non-Hispanic	31.5
Black alone	34.9
Asian alone	20.1
Hispanic (any race)	24.6
Some other race alone or in combination	33.2
DISABILITIES BY SEX	**PERCENT**
Male	19.8
Female	24.4

Source: Courtney-Long et al., 2015

About 27 million women in the US, or 24.4%, have disability, and this number is increasing. More than 50% of women older than 65 live with a disability. Women are more likely to have disability in the physical (31.6%) and mental (14.2%) domains. In contrast, men are more likely to have communication disability (12.8%). By functional type of disability, impaired mobility or mobility disability is the most frequently reported type in adults in the US (13.0%). Other types and their prevalence rates are cognitive disability (10.6%), inability to live independently (6.5%), impaired vision (4.6%), and self-care disability (3.6%) (Courtney-Long et al., 2015). The following sidebar presents a summary of facts about persons with disability.

SUMMARY OF FACTS ABOUT THE POPULATION OF PEOPLE WITH DISABILITY

- More than 61.4 million persons, or one in four (25.7%) noninstitutionalized adults in the US, have a disability (Okoro et al., 2018).
- More than 1 billion people (15% of the world's population) have one or more disabilities (The World Bank, 2020).
- Between 110 and 190 million (20%) of the world's total persons with disability experience significant limitations due to disability (The World Bank, 2020).
- Across all age groups, the prevalence of disability is higher in women than men (Okoro et al., 2018).
- The prevalence of disability and of each type of disability in the US is highest in American Indians/Alaska natives and lowest among Asians (Okoro et al., 2018).
- The prevalence of disability and each type of disability is higher among those who are poor than those who do not live in poverty (United Nations, 2018; Okoro et al., 2018).
- The percentage of people with disabilities living below the poverty level is twice that of people without disabilities (United Nations, 2018).
- Persons with disability are much less likely to be employed (19.1%) than those without disability (65.9%), and those who do work are more likely to work part time than those who do not have a disability (United Nations, 2018).
- The prevalence of disability and each type of disability is higher in the South compared to other regions of the US and is higher among those living in rural settings than urban settings (Okoro et al., 2018; Zhao, Okoro, Hsia, Garvin & Town, 2019).
- Adults with disability are four times as likely as those without disability to report fair or poor health (40.3% vs. 9.9%, respectively) (Krahn, Walker, & Correa-DeAraujo, 2015; United Nations, 2018).
- People with disability have shorter life expectancies and are at greater risk of co-morbid, secondary, and age-related health conditions and mental or psychological disorders than those without disability (United Nations, 2018).

continues

- People with disability have higher rates of obesity, hypertension, cardiovascular disease, lack of physical activity, falls-related injuries, and mood disorders such as depression than those without disability (United Nations, 2018).
- Persons with disability encounter greater barriers to healthcare than those who do not have a disability (United Nations, 2018).
- While persons with disability have higher rates of chronic disease than the general population, they are significantly less likely to receive preventive care and health screening (United Nations, 2018).
- Persons with disability are at increased risk for domestic or partner violence, physical assault, and sexual assault, with women and people with cognitive disabilities at highest risk (Krahn et al., 2015).
- Limited mobility is the most prevalent type of disability (13.7%), followed by cognitive disability (10.8%), impaired ability to live independently (6.8%), and impaired hearing (5.9%) (Okoro et al., 2018).

SUMMARY

Disability is a major issue that affects individuals, families, communities, and society as a whole. Lack of access for people with disability to services, support, and healthcare is a global concern that requires a global response. Although one in every four to five people across the globe lives with one or more disabilities, and many studies have pointed to inequities in both health and healthcare that affect those with disability, the topic of disability is one that is not well addressed by healthcare providers or healthcare professions' educational programs. It is important for healthcare professionals—all of whom *will* encounter people with disability in their roles as healthcare providers regardless of clinical setting—to be prepared to provide quality care so that those with disability can lead full, healthy lives.

REFERENCES

American Association on Intellectual and Developmental Disabilities. (2012). *User's guide to intellectual disability: definition, classification, and systems of support.* Silver Spring, MD: Author.

Americans with Disabilities Act of 1990, 42 U.S.C. § 12101 (1990).

Centers for Disease Control and Prevention. (n.d.-a). Developmental disabilities. Retrieved from https://www.cdc.gov/ncbddd/developmentaldisabilities/index.html

Centers for Disease Control and Prevention. (n.d.-b) Facts about intellectual disability. Retrieved from https://www.cdc.gov/ncbddd/developmentaldisabilities/facts-about-intellectual-disability.html

Centers for Disease Control and Prevention. (n.d.-c) Language and speech disorders in children. Retrieved from https://www.cdc.gov/ncbddd/childdevelopment/language-disorders.html

Centers for Disease Control and Prevention (n.d.-d) Vision loss: A public health issue. Retrieved from https://www.cdc.gov/visionhealth/basic_information/vision_loss.htm

Centers for Disease Control and Prevention. (n.d.-e) What is hearing loss in children? Retrieved from https://www.cdc.gov/ncbddd/hearingloss/facts.html

Centers for Disease Control and Prevention. (2011). Cognitive impairment: A call for action, now! Retrieved from https://www.cdc.gov/aging/pdf/cognitive_impairment/coglmp_poilicy_final.pdf

Centers for Medicare and Medicaid Services [CMS]. (2019). Modernizing health care to improve physical accessibility. https://www.cms.gov/About-CMS/Agency-Information/OMH/Downloads/OMH-Modernizing-Health-Care-Physical-Accessibility.pdf

Courtney-Long, E. A., Carroll, D. D., Zhang, Q. C., Stevens, A. C., Griffin-Blake, S., Armour, B. S., & Campbell, V. A. (2015). Prevalence of disability and disability type among adults – United States, 2013. *Morbidity and Mortality Weekly Report, 64*(29), 777–783. doi:10.15585/mmwr.MM6429a2

Iezzoni, L. I., Kurtz, S. G., & Rao, S. R. (2014). Trends in U.S. adult chronic disability rates over time. *Disability Health Journal, 7*(4), 402–412. doi:10.1016/j.dhjo.2014.05.007

Individuals with Disabilities Education Act, 42 U.S.C. § 18001 (1990).

Institute for Health Metrics and Evaluation. (2019). *Findings from the global burden of disease study 2017.* Seattle, WA: Author.

Institute of Medicine. (2007). *The future of disability in America.* Washington, D.C.: The National Academies Press.

International Council of Nurses. (2010). Prevention of disability and the care of people with disabilities [position statement]. Geneva, Switzerland: Author. Retrieved from http://www.icn.ch/publications/position-statements

Kirschner, K. L., & Curry, R. H. (2009). Educating health care professionals to care for patients with disabilities. *Journal of the American Medical Association, 302*(12), 1,334–1,335. doi:10.1001/jama.2009.1398

Krahn, G. L., Walker, D. K., & Correa-De-Araujo, R. (2015). Persons with disabilities as an unrecognized health disparity population. *American Journal of Public Health, 105,* S198–S206. doi:10.2105/AJPH.2014.302182

National Council on Disability. (2009). *The current state of health care for people with disabilities*. Washington, D.C.: Author.

National Institute of Neurological Disorders and Stroke. (2019). Spina bifida fact sheet. Retrieved from https://www.ninds.nih.gov/Disorders/Patient-Caregiver-Education/Fact-Sheets/Spina-Bifida-Fact-Sheet

National Institutes of Health. (n.d.). Intellectual and developmental disabilities. Retrieved from https://www.nichd.nih.gov/health/topics/idds/conditioninfo/default

National Institutes of Health. National Institute on Deafness and Other Communication Disorders. (2019). Specific language impairment. NIH publication No. 11-7751.

Office of the Surgeon General, National Institute of Child Health and Human Development, & Centers for Disease Control and Prevention. (2002). *Closing the gap: A national blueprint to improve the health of persons with mental retardation: Report of the Surgeon General's Conference on Health Disparities and Mental Retardation*. Washington, D.C.: US Department of Health and Human Services.

Office of the Surgeon General & Office on Disability. (2005). *The Surgeon General's call to action to improve the health and wellness of persons with disabilities*. Rockville, MD: Author.

Okoro, C. A., Hollis, N. D., Cyrus, A. C., & Griffin-Blake, S. (2018). Prevalence of disabilities and health care access by disability status and type among adults—United States, 2016. *Morbidity and Mortality Weekly Report, 67*(32), 882–887. doi: 10.15585/mmwr.mm6732a3

Patient Protection and Affordable Care Act, 42 U.S.C. § 18001. (2010).

Social Security Administration. (2020). *Red book*. Retrieved from https://www.ssa.gov/redbook/eng/definedisability.htm

United Nations. (2006). Convention on the Rights of Persons with Disabilities (CRPD). Retrieved from https://www.un.org/development/desa/disabilities/convention-on-the-rights-of-persons-with-disabilities.html

United Nations. (2018). *Disability and development report: Realizing the sustainable development goals by, for and with persons with disabilities*. New York, NY: Author.

United Nations. (2019). International day of persons with disabilities 3 December. Retrieved from https://www.un.org/en/observances/day-of-persons-with-disabilities/background

US Department of Education. (2018). Individuals with Disabilities Education Act (IDEA). Retrieved from https://sites.ed.gov/idea/regs/b/a/300.8

US Department of Health and Human Services. Office of Disease Prevention and Health Promotion. (2010). Disability and health. Retrieved from https://www.healthypeople.gov/2020/topics-objectives/topic/disability-and-health

World Health Organization. (2001). International classification of functioning, disability and health (ICF). Retrieved from https://www.who.int/classifications/icf/en/

World Health Organization. (2011). World report on disability. Retrieved from https://www.who.int/publications/i/item/world-report-on-disability

World Health Organization. (2016). Congenital anomalies. Retrieved from https://www.who.int/news-room/fact-sheets/detail/congenital-anomalies

World Health Organization. (2018). Disability and health. Retrieved from https://www.who.int/news-room/fact-sheets/detail/disability-and-health

2

THE ROLE OF SOCIAL DETERMINANTS OF HEALTH IN DISABILITY

INTRODUCTION

As noted in Chapter 1, healthcare received by people with disability, regardless of type of disability, is inferior to care received by those without disability. This lack of quality healthcare results in health inequities. These differences in the quality of healthcare, and in the health status of those with disability, are largely preventable. This chapter discusses the social determinants of health that play a role in these health inequities. It also highlights models of disability, explains the difference between disability and disabling conditions, addresses disability etiquette, and offers a brief history of disability and disability rights.

HEALTH INEQUITIES AND SOCIAL DETERMINANTS OF HEALTH

The term *health inequity*, or *health inequality*, refers to the inequitable and preventable burden of disease, disability, injury, or violence experienced by socially disadvantaged populations, and to the lack of opportunities for these populations to achieve optimal health (Braverman, 2014; World Health Organization [WHO], 2018).

The causes of these inequities are usually a lack of opportunities and unequal treatment, or discrimination, within the healthcare system (Krahn, Walker, & Correa-De-Araujo, 2015). This unequal treatment or discrimination is often a result of social and other determinants of health, such as the following:

- The physical and social environment
- The availability of health services
- Economic resources
- Social and political power

All these factors affect people's ability to obtain quality healthcare and achieve an optimal level of health (Krahn et al., 2015; National Academies of Sciences, Engineering, and Medicine, 2017; US Department of Health and Human Services [USDHHS], 2010, 2011).

> These social determinants—which are often influenced by policy decisions—are responsible for most health inequities.

Health inequity is often used to describe differences in health status or access to healthcare by members of different racial or ethnic groups or by people of different ages, genders, sexual orientations, immigration statuses, socioeconomic classes, and education levels. However, there are also serious health inequities due to disability status. These have a major impact on the well-being of people with disability. Further, people who face discrimination for other reasons (race, ethnicity, age, gender, sexual orientation, immigrant status, socioeconomic class, or education level) are at additional risk if they have a disability.

> Although disability status is a significant cause of health inequity, people with disability are often overlooked in discussions of social determinants of health.

HEALTH INEQUITIES VERSUS HEALTH DISPARITIES

The term *health disparities* is often used interchangeably with *health inequities* or *health inequalities* to describe differences in health status due to social injustice. This is incorrect, however. *Health disparities* are differences in health status that may or may not be a result of social injustice. For example, male infants generally weigh more than female infants at birth. This is considered a health disparity, not a health inequity.

Per the Healthy People 2020 initiative, social determinants of health of particular relevance to people with disability include the following (Krahn et al., 2015; USDHHS, 2010):

* Environmental barriers (often referred to as the *built environment*)

- Educational inequalities and lower levels of education
- Limited access to the internet
- Poverty or economic instability
- Limited access to employment opportunities and lower levels of employment
- Limited access to transportation
- Individual and behavioral factors
- Lack of information on health promotion
- Lack of access to healthcare, including preventive services

People with a disability are also more likely to encounter social barriers to accessing healthcare services and navigating the complex healthcare system. These barriers include the following (Centers for Disease Control and Prevention [CDC, CDC, n.d.-a., -b; WHO, 2018):

- Stigma associated with disability
- Myths and misconceptions about disability
- Lack of knowledge about disability
- Negative societal attitudes
- Negative attitudes on the part of healthcare professionals

Examples of health inequities that relate to disability include the following:

- Women with disability receive less screening for breast and cervical cancer than women without disability.
- Adolescents and adults with disability are less likely to be included in sex education programs.
- People with intellectual disability and pregnant women with disability are less likely than those without disability to be weighed during healthcare visits.

- People with disability are more susceptible to certain disorders, such as pressure ulcers, osteoporosis, and urinary tract infections.

- People with disability are more vulnerable to secondary conditions, co-morbid conditions, and age-related conditions than people without disability.

- People with disability engage in higher levels of behaviors that put their health at risk than people without disability.

- Conditions that might be a mere inconvenience or annoyance to someone without a disability can have major health consequences for someone with a disability.

- People with disability have greater unmet healthcare needs than people without disability.

> Health inequity does not suggest that having a disability means that a person cannot be healthy or that disability is equivalent to poor health. It simply means that people with disability have more unmet health-related needs than people without disability.

Because of these and other health inequities, people with disability are significantly more likely to report fair or poor health than those without disability (40.3% versus 9.9%) (Krahn et al., 2015; United Nations, 2018). They also experience higher rates of premature death (WHO, 2018).

MODELS OF DISABILITY

Several models of disability have been developed over the years to address health inequities, including inadequate healthcare as well as limited access to healthcare, education, and employment opportunities for individuals with disability. The purpose of these models is to foster understanding of the concept of disability and to identify assumptions, concerns, and views about disability and the nature of the human experience of having a disability. These models provide definitions of disability, identify guidelines for action (including

---

policy change), and foster the examination of one's values (Retief & Letšosa, 2018; Smart, 2004; Smith & Bundon, 2017).

This section discusses several (but not all) models of disability. These include the following:

- The medical model of disability

- The rehabilitation model of disability

- The social model of disability

- The human rights model of disability

- The interface model of disability

- Other models of disability

These are discussed in the following sections to illustrate how different models influence the attitudes and perceptions of healthcare providers, and how this in turn affects the health and well-being of people with disability.

Note that not all of these models are recommended for adoption. This is because some of these models do not recognize the autonomy of people with disability. Preferred models promote health; disavow discrimination; recognize the ability of those with disability to identify, communicate, and make decisions about their health-related needs; and acknowledge the condition or disorder that has resulted in disability.

Learning about models of disability affects how healthcare providers, including nurses, view and interact with people with disability, both in their care and in decision-making about their care.

THE MEDICAL MODEL OF DISABILITY

The medical model of disability, sometimes referred to as the individual model of disability, has historically defined disability for healthcare or medical professionals. This model is based on the principle that disability is a disease or medical problem that impairs the performance of an activity.

This model rests on the view that people with disability are not and cannot be "normal" due to the impairment. Further, it does not address the role that a person's environment has in the disability. That is, the model situates the impairment within the affected person, ignoring societal attitudes and structures that oppress people with disability. Finally, this model considers disability to be a personal tragedy for the individual and family and something that needs to be "fixed." In other words, it views individuals with disability as tragic (Retief & Letšosa, 2018) and sees those who "overcome" their disability as heroic or inspirational.

The medical model of disability has been criticized because it is based on the views of able-bodied medical professionals who may see people with disability as defective or "not normal." With this model, healthcare providers are seen as the experts or authorities on a person's disability, and curing the disability is the focus of medical management. If curing the disability is not possible, then the goal is to promote adjustment or behavior change on the part of the person with the disability.

The disability community believes the medical model promotes passivity and dependency and promotes a negative view of those with disability (Retief & Letšosa, 2018; Smart, 2004; Smith & Bundon, 2017).

THE REHABILITATION MODEL OF DISABILITY

The rehabilitation model of disability is based on and shares the same views as the medical model. In this model, the healthcare provider—usually a rehabilitation specialist—is considered to be the expert who can "fix" the problem or disability for the patient, while those with disability are viewed as having failed to work hard enough to overcome their disability. The criticisms of this model are similar to those of the medical model.

THE SOCIAL MODEL OF DISABILITY

This model, developed by disability activists in response to the limitations of the medical model, rejects the notion that disability and health are mutually exclusive. Instead, this model sees disability as resulting from society's failure to accommodate the needs of people with disability. In other words, the model—along with variations of it in the UK (also called the social model of disability)—considers disability to be a social construct. Some variations of this model go further, viewing disability as a result of oppression by an unaccommodating society. Under this model, societal change through political activism is viewed as the solution to disability.

Although this model has empowered many people with disability, it has been criticized as limiting and for ignoring the contributions of functional impairment to disability (Retief & Letšosa , 2018; Shakespeare, 2013; Smith & Bundon, 2017). This model is also discussed in Chapter 9.

THE HUMAN RIGHTS MODEL OF DISABILITY

This model focuses on the rights of people with disability to be free from discrimination and to have access all the same services and opportunities as those without disability. An example of the human rights model of disability, the United Nations Convention on the Rights of Persons with Disabilities (CRPD), has identified eight important underlying principles (United Nations, 2012):

- Respect for the inherent dignity, individual autonomy (including the freedom to make one's own choices), and independence of people

- Nondiscrimination

- Full and effective inclusion and participation in society

- Respect for difference and acceptance of people with disability as part of human diversity and humanity

- Equality of opportunity

- Accessibility

- Equality between men and women

- Respect for the evolving capacities of children with disability and their right to preserve their identities

The human rights model holds that all policies and laws should be designed with the involvement and input of people with disability and calls for the inclusion of disability in all aspects of political action.

THE INTERFACE MODEL OF DISABILITY

The interface model is not a fully developed model. However, it has merit because of its focus on the interaction or intersection of the disabling condition and its disabling effects. The intent of the model, developed by a nurse with a disability (Goodall, 1995), is to promote care designed to empower rather than care that fosters or increases dependency. The model encourages the view that people with disability are responsible people who are capable of functioning despite the presence of a disability. This model can serve as a basis for nurses and other healthcare professionals to advocate for the elimination of discrimination and removal of barriers to healthcare. The model also provides direction for examination and for the elimination of practices that result in the view of disability as an abnormal state.

OTHER MODELS OF DISABILITY

Several other models of disability exist, and others are evolving. Existing models include the following:

- **The Nagi disablement model:** This early model of disability defined terms that now appear in the WHO International

Classification of Functioning, Disability and Health (ICF), which is used to create a common language for describing and understanding health and health status.

- **The charity model of disability:** One of the oldest models of disability, the charity model views people with disability as tragic and as objects of pity.

- **The economic model:** This model approaches disability from the perspective of the contributions of people with disability to society and their ability to be employed in meaningful work.

- **The social relational model of disability:** This model views disability as a manifestation of social relationships between people and the social forces and structures that result in disablism (Retief & Letšosa, 2018; Smith & Bundon, 2017). It addresses criticisms of the social model by accounting for the lived experience of people with disability who face discrimination, oppression, or abuse from others (*disablism*) and who live with impairment.

DISABILITY VERSUS DISABLING CONDITION

Many healthcare providers understand in detail the pathophysiology and the physical, psychological, mental, or behavioral features of a specific disabling condition but fail to appreciate its impact on a person's daily life and future, or its implications on that person's access to healthcare. For example, a healthcare provider might understand the physical effects of a spinal cord injury at the seventh thoracic vertebrae on a person's ability to move or turn without assistance and to control bowel and bladder function. However, the healthcare provider might not appreciate the consequences of the injury on the individual's ability to participate in usual activities of daily living, carry out self-care, attend school, work at a satisfying job, establish relationships with others, have satisfying sexual relationships, and have and raise children.

To be of genuine assistance to those with disability, and to ensure these people receive the high quality of healthcare they need and deserve, healthcare providers must understand the day-to-day lives and experiences of people with disability. Simply knowing about disabling conditions is not enough. They must understand disability and all that the term implies. Conveying this essential knowledge is the focus and objective of this book.

PREFERRED DISABILITY LANGUAGE AND ETIQUETTE

Many people, aware of past discrimination against those with disability and of a general lack of sensitivity in interacting with them, are concerned about what language to use when referring to people with disability. In general, the use of person-first language is accepted and preferred. An example of person-first language is "the person with a disability." In contrast, "the disabled person" or simply "the disabled" is *not* first-person language. Non-first-person language should be avoided. Just as one would not (or should not) refer to someone with diabetes as "the diabetic," one should not refer to a person with disability as "the disabled."

Other differences may exist from one group of people with disability to another. For example, there are differences in preferences among people who have hearing loss. Those who have been deaf since birth and use sign language often prefer "Deaf" over "deaf." Moreover, many of these people do not see themselves as having a disability; rather, they consider themselves and others who are Deaf as part of a separate culture or community.

When interacting with people with a disability, it is important to ask them what they prefer. For example, some people might prefer *not* to be described by any wording that uses the term disability, while others might have specific preferences. It is important to avoid making assumptions, to find out what each person prefers, and to respect that person's preferences (United Spinal Association, 2015).

Table 2.1 presents general tips about interacting with people with disability. More specific examples of appropriate ways to interact with people with disability are included in chapters on specific categories of disability.

TABLE 2.1   STRATEGIES FOR INTERACTING WITH PEOPLE WITH DISABILITY

Communication strategies	Ask about the person's preferred means of communication (e.g., writing; sign language, interpreter, other).
	Ensure that the preferred method of communication is available and made known to other healthcare professionals.
	Direct all communication to the person with a disability rather than to others accompanying that person.
	Use person-first language.
	Treat adults with disability as responsible people who can communicate their needs and make decisions about care.
	Respect the person's privacy just as you would anyone else's.
	When giving instructions or directions, be specific.
Strategies for interacting with people with mobility impairment	Do not assume that a person with a mobility or other physical limitation needs help. Ask first.
	Do not assume that a person who uses a mobility device is unable to participate in physical activities.
	Be sensitive about physical contact without asking first. Avoid touching mobility devices (wheelchairs, crutches, canes, walkers, etc.), as these are part of the person's physical space and critical to mobility and independence.
	Sit at eye level when interacting with wheelchair users.

Strategies for interacting with people with com- munication impairment	Do not assume that someone with a communication disability has a limited ability to understand what is being said or to make decisions.
	Do not interrupt people who are speaking, cut short what they are saying, or finish their sentence.
	Do not pretend that you understand what someone has said when you don't. Ask people to repeat themselves.
Strategies for interacting with people with sensory impairment	Ask a person who has vision or hearing impairment how they would like you to communicate with them.
	Ensure that preferred accommodations are available.
	If an interpreter is used to assist with communication, talk directly to the person with a disability rather than to the inter- preter.
	Use normal volume when speaking with someone with sensory impairment. Shouting is not necessary and may make it more difficult to be understood.
	Do not exaggerate mouth movements in an effort to be under- stood. Doing so may make it more difficult for someone who speech/lip reads to understand.
Strategies for interacting with people with cognitive impairment	Have conversations with people with cognitive impairment in a quiet environment without distractions.
	Speak to the person in clear sentences using simple words and concrete concepts.
	Treat adults with cognitive impairment as adults.
	Do not treat or speak to an adult with cognitive impartment using words or tone of voice that you would use when speaking to an infant or young child.
	Assume that people with cognitive impairment can communi- cate their needs rather than rely on others accompanying them.
	Use nonwritten means (e.g., pictures or figures) to communi- cate if that approach works better for the person with cognitive impairment.
	Allow adequate time for a person with cognitive impairment to understand what is being said.
	Respect the privacy of the person with cognitive impairment just as you would anyone else's privacy.

A BRIEF HISTORY OF DISABILITY AND DISABILITY RIGHTS

Although global attention on disability has grown in recent years, disability is not new. Rather, it is an ancient topic—one that existed long before people were able to record how people with disability were treated in ancient societies. We do know, however, that people with disability were often seen as victims of a curse or punishment from God for their own behavior or that of their relatives and ancestors. Disability was also seen as a failure, deformity, or defect of the person. (Smeltzer, Mariani, & Meakim, 2017).

> Oppression and discrimination against people with disability can be traced back to biblical times, if not earlier.

People who had types of disabilities that are strongly associated with stigma—for example, psychiatric mental disability, intellectual or cognitive disability, and certain types of neurological disability—were often kept hidden from others. Their existence was considered shameful to their families, and they were considered a drain on society. Often, people with disability were feared and ostracized or were objects of pity. Many were institutionalized in almshouses or asylums. Even today, people with certain disabilities in some societies are abandoned to die or are killed because of the fears and superstitions of others.

Literature has often portrayed people with disability as having lower economic and social value than those without disability. Those with disability have also often been portrayed as beggars or thieves. There is some basis for these depictions, however. In some societies, adults and children with disability were forced to beg on the street because they had no other means of supporting themselves. Family members hoped that pity for the person begging would result in more money received.

> Some people with disability have been used as court jesters to entertain others or as oddities in circuses and freak shows.

Dramatic shifts in how those with disability were treated occurred during the late eighteenth and nineteenth centuries. Schools and institutions were established to house those with disability. However, although they provided some education, these schools and institutions were segregated and often isolated.

Tumultuous times in history have not been kind to people with disability. Personal histories and other documents reveal that during the Nazi era in pre–World War II Germany, people with disability were the first victims of euthanasia programs undertaken to eliminate those who were deemed "unfit" and "undesirable." Even before the Nazi regime, however, people with disability who resided in German psychiatric institutions were subject to mistreatment, sterilization, experiments, and even death.

Such discrimination against people with disability was not confined to Germany. Marriage and childbearing by people with disability were discouraged if not prohibited in the United States and elsewhere. In 1927, Justice Oliver Wendell Holmes of the US Supreme Court ruled that compulsory sterilization of the "unfit"—that is, people with disability—was constitutional. In ruling that a young woman who was erroneously thought to have an intellectual disability could be forcibly sterilized, Justice Holmes famously stated, "Three generations of imbeciles are enough" (Fries, 2017; U.S. Holocaust Memorial Museum, 2018).

Because of these and many other reprehensible practices over the years, disability activists worldwide have made many efforts to improve the plight of people with disability. These activists have sought to ensure that people with disability are treated in humane and dignified ways and that they have access to the same opportunities and resources as people without disability. As the civil rights movement in the United States grew to address racial inequities, disability rights activists saw an opportunity to advocate for legislation to end the centuries-old discrimination against, negative stereotypes about, and attitudes toward those with disability that served as barriers against their full participation in society. Disability became an issue that had implications in terms of health, society, and policy.

Several laws were passed to support equal employment, income, housing, and transportation for people with disability. However, the Americans with Disabilities Act (ADA) of 1990 was the first comprehensive civil rights law designed to prevent exclusion and discrimination based on disability status. The ADA addresses the rights of people with disability in many parts of society and was designed to meet four specific goals for this population:

- Equal employment opportunities

- Full participation in the community

- Independent living

- Economic self-sufficiency

Although the ADA mandated these changes, it did not guarantee that strategies to accomplish these goals would be implemented. So, although the ADA has increased access to healthcare for people with disability, progress has been slower than desired (Peacock, Iezzoni, & Harkin, 2015).

One persistent and current issue pertaining to people with disability is quality of life. Others have often viewed the quality of life of people with disability as poor, even though the only person who can gauge the quality of life of a person with a disability is the person with the disability. In recent years, the question of whether the quality of life of people with severe disability is good or even acceptable has been raised in discussions about assisted suicide. The view of disability activists, advocates, and others is that assisted suicide legislation devalues and even targets people with disability, even though they are not mentioned specifically. Potential legislation often defines a person as terminally ill and eligible for assisted suicide if that person is likely to die within six months without treatment. The concern of disability advocates and activists is that this definition includes many people with disability, who, with proper treatment, can live very satisfying lives for decades. They view the wording of such legislation as license for family members or others to coerce those with disability to end their lives (Center for Disability Rights, n.d.).

INSURANCE AND OTHER FINANCIAL RESOURCES

Healthcare of children and adults with disability is often complex and usually very expensive. This makes a lack of insurance and other financial resources a major barrier to obtaining healthcare and a major social determinant of health for this population. Fortunately, there are a number of financial resources available to individuals with disability as well as for families with children with disability.

Many of the financial resources available to individuals with disability and their families are funded by the federal government and administered by the states. For example, the Centers for Medicare and Medicaid Services (CMS) partners with states and national organizations to ensure that persons with disability and chronic disease receive access to health insurance and healthcare information. Medicare and Medicaid are examples of programs operated and funded by different parts of the government. Each one serves different groups.

In the US, health insurance is often tied to employment. So, for many individuals with disability who lack employment or are employed less than full time, these financial resources are especially important.

Individuals with disability and families with children with disability may need to be referred to social workers or financial advisors with knowledge about the complex programs that are available. Programs and benefits often differ by state, as do waiting periods for eligibility and criteria for disability. Individuals with disability must be evaluated and provide considerable documentation to ensure that they meet the definitions of disability used by these programs. This can be a time-consuming and frustrating process for those with disability and their families; therefore, they are encouraged to initiate the process sooner than later.

The implementation of the Patient Protection and Affordable Care Act (also known as the ACA or Obamacare) has had significant positive implications for adults and children with disability. In the past, the presence of a preexisting condition (e.g., intellectual or developmental disability, other types of disability, chronic disease, and so on) often resulted in individuals with disability being refused insurance or being charged more than those without disability. The passage of the ACA brought about three important changes:

- Insurers are no longer permitted to deny coverage due to disability or other preexisting conditions.

- People cannot lose or be denied the right to renew their insurance simply because they become sick or develop a disability.

- Insurance companies are prohibited from charging premiums based on health conditions—meaning that people cannot be charged more simply because they have a disability (USDHHS, n.d.).

The following are programs relevant to healthcare and well-being of adults and children with disability and their families:

- **Medicaid:** This state and federal program provides health insurance for adults with disability as well as for people with a low income. Adults under 65 years of age and children with disability since birth or an acquired disability because of illness or trauma are eligible for Medicaid. In addition to covering costs associated with acute healthcare, Medicaid covers costs of long-term care for older adults and people of all ages with disability in nursing homes and in the community (Medicaid.gov, n.d.-c).

- **Medicare:** This state and federal program provides health insurance for people who are 65 years of age and older, certain younger people with disability, and individuals with end-stage renal disease. Medicare covers costs of certain hospital, nursing home, home health, physician, and community-based services. These healthcare services do not have to be related to the individual's disability to be covered. Different parts of Medicare cover specific services:

- **Medicare Part A (hospital insurance):** This covers inpatient hospital stays, care in a skilled nursing facility, hospice care, and some home healthcare.

- **Medicare Part B (medical insurance):** This covers fees for physicians and other healthcare providers, outpatient care, mental health services, and certain home health visits, medical supplies, and preventive health services.

- **Medicare Part D (prescription drug coverage):** This helps cover the cost of prescription drugs, including many recommended shots or vaccines.

Medicare Part C, also known as Medicare Advantage, does not provide support for individuals with disability in most states and is included here merely for completeness. It allows most beneficiaries—except individuals with disability in most states—to sign up for a managed care program for their Medicare Part A and Part B benefits. People who enroll in Part C pay a fee for managed care enrollment (Medicare.gov, n.d.).

- **Medicaid waivers:** Most states have developed Medicaid waivers, also referred to as home and community-based services (HCBS) waivers, to allow children who depend on technology (e.g., a ventilator) to receive long-term care in the home and to continue to receive financial support for care (Betz & Nehring, 2010; Medicaid.gov, n.d.-b).

- **Children's Health Insurance Program (CHIP):** This program is funded jointly by states and the federal government. CHIP provides low-cost health coverage to children. Each state offers CHIP coverage and works closely with its state Medicaid program, based on federal requirements. Coverage may differ by state (Medicaid.gov, n.d.-a).

- **Social Security Disability Insurance (SSDI):** This program provides payment to individuals with disability who are unable to work because of their disability. To be eligible, an individual must have worked for a specific number of years and contributed to Social Security. The requirements differ by age (Social Security Administration, 2019).

- **Supplemental Security Income (SSI):** This provides a federal cash assistance program for older adults and for people with disability who have low levels of income. SSI makes monthly payments to people with low income and limited resources who are 65 years of age or older, are blind, or have another type of disability. Children younger than 18 years of age qualify if they have a medical condition or combination of conditions that results in marked and severe functional limitations and if their income and family income and resources fall within the eligibility limit. The amount of cash payment varies by state (Social Security Administration, 2020).

This brief overview of the many resources and agencies available to ensure that individuals with disability have appropriate financial resources reveals the complexity of the task that families and those with disability must take on to obtain those resources. An understanding of the complexity is important for nurses and other healthcare professionals so they can be supportive and assist in the process when possible.

SUMMARY

Many factors affect the lives, health, and well-being of individuals with disability. Health inequities that occur with disability are often due to social determinants of health. Many people with disability experience multiple inequities that compound the barriers they encounter in their desire to obtain quality healthcare.

Multiple models of disability have been developed over time to recognize the issues and barriers facing people with a disability. In some cases, the models provide direction to identify general solutions for addressing those barriers. For healthcare providers, including nurses, to provide quality care to people with disability, they need to grasp more than the underlying physiological, psychological, or mental causes or consequences of disability. They must have a grasp of the day-to-day lives of people striving to overcome barriers that affect their experiences and their ability to obtain healthcare.

Because of the importance of communication in all healthcare situations and settings—and in providers' interactions with patients, clients, and family members—healthcare providers must be sensitive to the effect of their verbal and nonverbal communication on people with disability. It is critically important that the preferences of people with disability and their family members be honored. It is also critical that those with disability are not ignored in their interactions with healthcare providers. Too often, providers find it more convenient to talk around the person with disability, which is both demeaning and insensitive.

It is important to understand the history of disability so that we do not repeat mistakes of the past. Although negative treatment of people with disability is unacceptable to most people, society—and healthcare professionals within society—harbors more subtle forms of discrimination and bias. Understanding the history of disability promotes an examination of behaviors and biases that affect people with disability. (Note that issues of bias in healthcare affecting those with disability are addressed in further detail in other chapters of this book.)

REFERENCES

Betz, C. L., & Nehring, W. M. (2010). *Nursing care for individuals with intellectual and developmental disabilities: An integrated approach*. Baltimore, MD: Brookes Publishing.

Braverman, P. (2014). What are health disparities and health equity? We need to be clear. *Public Health Reports, 129*(Suppl 2), 5–8. doi:10.1177/00333549141291S203

Center for Disability Rights. (n.d.). Assisted suicide kills people with disabilities. Retrieved from http://cdrnys.org/assisted-suicide

Centers for Disease Control and Prevention. (n.d.-a). Common barriers to participation experienced by people with disabilities. Retrieved from https://www.cdc.gov/ncbddd/disabilityandhealth/disability-barriers.html

Centers for Disease Control and Prevention. (n.d.-b). Disability and health inclusion strategies. Retrieved from https://www.cdc.gov/ncbddd/disabilityandhealth/disability-strategies.html

Fries, K. (2017). The Nazis' first victims were the disabled. *The New York Times.* Retrieved from https://www.nytimes.com/2017/09/13/opinion/nazis-holocaust-disabled.html

Goodall, C. J. (1995). Is disability any business of nurse education? *Nurse Education Today, 15*(5), 323–327. doi:10.1016/s0260-6917(95)80003-4

Krahn, G. L., Walker, D. K., & Correa-De-Araujo, R. (2015). Persons with disabilities as an unrecognized health disparity population. *American Journal of Public Health, 105*(Suppl 2), S198–S206. doi:10.2105/AJPH.2014.302182

Medicaid.gov. (n.d.-a). Children's Health Insurance Program (CHIP). Retrieved from https://www.medicaid.gov/chip/index.html

Medicaid.gov. (n.d.-b). Home and community-based services 1915(c). Retrieved from https://www.medicaid.gov/medicaid/home-community-based-services/home-community-based-services-authorities/home-community-based-services-1915c/index.html

Medicaid.gov. (n.d.-c) Medicaid. Retrieved from https://www.medicaid.gov/medicaid/index.html

Medicaid.gov. (n.d.-d) National Medicaid & CHIP program information Retrieved from https://www.medicaid.gov/medicaid/national-medicaid-chip-program-information/index.html

Medicare.gov. (n.d.) What Medicare covers. https://www.medicare.gov/what-medicare-covers

National Academies of Sciences, Engineering, and Medicine. (2017). *Communities in action: Pathways to health equity.* Washington, D.C.: The National Academies Press. https://doi.org/10.17226/24624

Peacock, G., Iezzoni, L. I., & Harkin, T. R. (2015). Health for Americans with disabilities—25 years after the ADA. *New England Journal of Medicine, 373*(1), 892–893. doi:10.1056/NEJMp1508854

Retief, R., & Letšosa, R. (2018). Models of disability: A brief overview. *Theological Studies, 74*(1), a475.

Shakespeare, T. (2013). The social model of disability. In L. J. Davis (Ed.), *The disability studies reader*, 4th ed. New York, NY: Routledge Press.

Smart, J. (2004). Models of disability: The juxtaposition of biology and social construction. In T. F. Riggar & D. R. Maki (Eds.), *Handbook of rehabilitation counseling* (pp. 25–49). New York, NY: Springer Publishing Co.

Smeltzer, S. C., Mariani, B., & Meakim, C. (2017). Brief historical view of disability and related legislation. Retrieved from http://www.nln.org/docs/default-source/professional-development-programs/ace-series/brief-history-of-disability.pdf?sfvrsn=6

Smith, B., & Bundon, A. (2017). Disability models: Explaining and understanding disability sport in different ways. In I. Brittain & A. Beacom (Eds.), *The Palgrave handbook of Paralympic studies* (pp. 15–34). London, UK: Palgrave.

Social Security Administration (2019). Disability benefits. Retrieved from https://www.ssa.gov/pubs/EN-05-10029.pdf

Social Security Administration (2020). Benefits for children with disabilities. Retrieved from https://www.ssa.gov/pubs/EN-05-10026.pdf

United Nations. (2012). *Convention on the Rights of Persons with Disabilities training guide*. New York, NY: United Nations.

United Nations (2018). UN flagship report on disability and development: Realization of the sustainable development goals, for and with persons with disabilities. NY: United Nations.

United Spinal Association. (2015). *Disability etiquette: Interacting with people with disabilities*. Retrieved from http://unitedspinal.org/disability-etiquette/

United States Holocaust Memorial Museum. (2018). *Nazi persecution of the disabled: Murder of the "unfit."* Retrieved from https://www.ushmm.org/information/exhibitions/online-exhibitions/special-focus/nazi-persecution-of-the-disabled/patricia-heberer-describes-nazi-public-health-strategies

US Department of Health and Human Services. (n.d.) What is the Affordable Care Act? https://www.hhs.gov/healthcare/about-the-aca/index.html

US Department of Health and Human Services. (2010). Healthy People 2020. Retrieved from https://www.cdc.gov/nchs/healthy_people/hp2020.htm

US Department of Health and Human Services. (2011). Healthy People 2010 Final Review. Retrieved from https://www.cdc.gov/nchs/data/hpdata2010/hp2010_final_review.pdf

World Health Organization. (2016). World health statistics 2016. Monitoring health for the SDGs. Retrieved from https://www.who.int/gho/publications/world_health_statistics/2016/en/

World Health Organization. (2018). Disability and health. Retrieved from https://www.who.int/news-room/fact-sheets/detail/disability-and-health

3
STRATEGIES TO ADDRESS BARRIERS TO HEALTHCARE FOR PEOPLE WITH DISABILITY

INTRODUCTION

As discussed in Chapter 1 and Chapter 2, people with disability often experience inadequate healthcare. As a result, they are at high risk for chronic conditions, poor quality of life, and increased morbidity and mortality. Causes of inadequate healthcare for this population have been attributed to many barriers that affect healthcare access. Nurses and other healthcare professionals must be aware of these barriers and either take steps to eliminate them (when possible) or work around them until they can be removed entirely.

The social determinants of health (refer to Chapter 2) are just some factors that affect access to healthcare for this population. There are also generic barriers that affect this population as a whole. The Centers for Disease Control and Prevention (CDC) describes these barriers as factors in an individual's environment that, through their absence or presence, limit functioning and create disability. They are as follows (CDC, n.d.-a):

- A physical environment that is not accessible

- A lack of assistive technology (assistive, adaptive, and rehabilitative devices)

- Negative attitudes toward disability and people with disability

- Services, systems, and policies that are either nonexistent or hinder the involvement of all people with a health condition in all areas of life

Experts identify five major categories of barriers. These categories are as follows:

- Attitudinal barriers

- Communication barriers

- Structural and physical barriers

- Programmatic barriers

- Transportation barriers

All these barriers are related. Even if only one category of barrier currently exists, that single barrier can cause other barriers. Moreover, addressing one type of barrier may have little effect on access to healthcare if other barriers are not also addressed. For example, even if physical barriers are removed, attitudinal barriers in the form of negative attitudes of healthcare professionals toward those with disability might remain. Finally, barriers often result in a negative snowball effect. For instance, the existence of physical or structural barriers can cause people with disability to be dependent on others, which in turn limits their participation in everyday life (World Health Organization [WHO], 2011).

ATTITUDINAL BARRIERS

The most difficult barriers to overcome are *attitudinal barriers*. These describe the negative attitudes of others, including healthcare professionals, toward people with disability. Examples of attitudinal barriers in healthcare include the following:

- Negative attitudes toward people with disability, resulting in stereotyping, bias, stigma, prejudice, and discrimination

- A lack of knowledge about the abilities and strengths of people with disability

- The assumption that people with disability are dependent, unaware of or uninterested in events around them, and unable to make decisions or otherwise participate in life activities

- The belief that all health issues that affect people with disability are due to their disability

- The failure to recognize, prevent, and treat common health issues that affect people with and without disability

- The assumption that the quality of life of people with disability is poor

Negative attitudes are often due to implicit or unconscious biases, which may be triggered without our even being aware of them. They result in attitudes about and preferences for others based on factors such as age, gender, race, ethnicity, national origin, socioeconomic status, sexual orientation, religion, body weight, and disability status (American Bar Association Commission on Disability Rights, 2019).

> Lack of contact with and lack of knowledge about others—in this case, people with disability—tend to reinforce the negative attitudes that we hold.

Implicit biases generally reflect our personal experiences; the attitudes of people we grew up with; the attitudes of our friends, acquaintances, and broader community; our culture; the media; and books and movies. We tend to harbor negative attitudes toward those who are different from us, who do not belong to the same groups as we do, or who do not share our characteristics. Consequences of implicit bias can include stereotyping, prejudice, and discriminatory behaviors or actions—although we may be unaware that we are exhibiting these behaviors or taking these actions.

Studies show that the negative attitudes of healthcare professionals and students toward people with disability do not differ significantly from the attitudes of society at large and in some cases are even worse (Tervo, Palmer, & Redinius, 2004). Further, health professionals and society at large tend to view people with certain disabilities more negatively than those with other disabilities. For example, people with intellectual or cognitive disabilities and those with psychiatric or

> Most calls to improve the healthcare of people with disability (refer to Chapter 1) have identified the need to include disability content and to increase the attention on disability in health professions curricula. Movement in that direction, however, has been slow.

mental health disabilities are viewed more negatively than people with physical disabilities (Pelleboer-Gunnink, Van Oorsouw, Van Weeghel, & Embregts, 2017).

A lack of attention to disability in the curricula of most health professions education (nursing, medicine, dentistry, and others) contributes to the negative attitudes of healthcare professionals toward people with disability. So, too, does a lack of opportunities for students in those professions to interact with people with diverse types of disabilities.

CONSEQUENCES OF ATTITUDINAL BARRIERS

The negative attitudes of healthcare professionals toward people with disability can have significant consequences. For example:

- Healthcare providers who believe that people with disability make no contribution to society will likely provide low-quality care or no care at all.

- Healthcare providers who believe that women with disability are (or should be) sexually inactive—or that they have no right to bear children—will likely make women with disability extremely uncomfortable during interactions with them. They might even provide substandard care to women with disability, refuse to provide reproductive healthcare to pregnant women with disability, or withhold information from women with disability about caring for their infants.

- Healthcare providers who believe that people with disability are incapable of making informed decisions might determine what care and treatment are warranted for patients with disability without consulting them, without offering any explanation, and without proposing treatment options.

The healthcare providers in these examples would likely be unaware of their negative attitudes and biases, and unaware of the discriminatory and prejudicial practices and behaviors that resulted.

STRATEGIES TO ADDRESS ATTITUDINAL BARRIERS

Strategies for healthcare professionals and educators to address attitudinal barriers include the following:

- Providing students with firsthand experiences interacting with people with disability during medical, nursing, and dental school (Shakespeare & Kleine, 2013; Symons, Morley, McGuigan, & Akl, 2014; Woodard, Havercamp, Zwygart, & Perkins, 2012)

- Including standardized patients with actual disability in health professions education (Long-Bellil et al., 2011; Smeltzer et al., 2018; Vest et al., 2016)

- Including people with disability on the educational team

Including people with disability on the educational team conveys that people with disability are experts on their disability. It also increases students' comfort interacting with people with disability and enables them to ask questions that they may otherwise be reluctant to ask about their disability and their daily lives. Finally, it provides an authentic learning experience and helps prevent stereotyping that often occurs when people pretend to have a disability for educational purposes. This practice should be avoided by inclusion of individuals with actual disability.

- Modeling positive behaviors, including communication, when interacting with people with disability

- Educating healthcare professions students about the health issues experienced by people with disability and the need to provide them with the same quality of healthcare, including health promotion and preventive screening, that is provided to others

- Educating people without knowledge or exposure to people with disability

- Not ignoring others' negative behaviors toward people with disability

Because of the tenacity of lifelong mindsets, strategies to address negative attitudes must be multiple, persistent, and repeated over time.

US FEDERAL LEGISLATION ON THE RIGHTS OF PEOPLE WITH DISABILITY

Healthcare professionals and organizations should be aware of national policy and legislation that protects the rights of people with disability and ensures that they are included in all aspects of society, including healthcare. Knowledge of the legal rights of these individuals helps ensure the provision of quality healthcare for this population now and in the future. Several of the most relevant federal laws are described briefly here (Bersani & Lyman, 2009; Institute of Medicine, 2007):

Section 504 of the Rehabilitation Act of 1973: This federal law protects people from discrimination based on disability by employers and organizations that receive financial assistance from federal departments or agencies. Section 504 of the Rehabilitation Act forbids organizations and employers from denying people with disability an equal opportunity to receive program benefits and services. Further, the act defines the rights of individuals with disability to participate in, and have access to, program benefits and services.

The Americans with Disabilities Act (ADA) of 1990: The ADA (and the ADA Amendments Act of 2008, discussed in the next bullet) protects the civil rights of people with disability and seeks to eliminate discrimination against them. Although there is further progress to be made, the ADA has helped to remove or reduce many barriers for people with disability. The ADA has also expanded opportunities for people with disability by changing perceptions and increasing participation of people with disability in community life. Specific areas identified in the ADA as guaranteed for people with disability include employment and public accommodations (e.g., at restaurants, hotels, theaters, doctors' offices, pharmacies, stores, museums, libraries, parks, private schools, and daycare centers). The ADA also requires that transportation, state and local government agencies, and telecommunications (e.g., telephones, televisions, and computers) be accessible to people with disability.

ADA Amendments Act (ADAAA) of 2008: This law was enacted to restore the original intent of the ADA after several Supreme Court decisions that limited the rights of people with disability. The ADAAA increased the number of people protected by the ADA and other nondiscrimination laws by broadening the law and redefining disability.

Patient Protection and Affordable Care Act (ACA) of 2010: This law increased healthcare choices and protection for people with disability. It also allowed for new healthcare options for long-term support and services; improved Medicaid home- and community-based services; increased access to high-quality and affordable healthcare for many people with disability; and enabled accessible preventive screening equipment. In addition, it designated disability as a demographic category to establish the inclusion of people with disability in the US census and in national studies. This will improve data about this population that have been missing from many governmental and other reports.

A CAUTION AGAINST DISABILITY SIMULATIONS

Disability simulations (or disability experiences) have been suggested and implemented as a strategy to increase the understanding of nondisabled people about disability. In a disability simulation, students might be placed in wheelchairs, or their hands and feet might be restrained to simulate a loss of mobility; they might be given opaque glasses or blindfolded to simulate vision loss; or their hearing might be modified to simulate hearing impairment.

People with disability and disability advocates caution that these simulations do not have long-lasting positive effects on learners and do not provide a realistic view of living with a disability. In some cases, after participating in such simulations, students indicated that they did not think having a disability was "so bad." In others, students left with a false sense and negative view of what living with a disability would be like (VanPuymbrouck, Heffron, Sheth, The, & Lee, 2017). Other negative outcomes include a lack of improved attitudes about interacting with people with disability, an undermining of efforts to improve the integration of people with disability, and increased stereotyping (Nario-Redmond, Gospodinov, & Cobb, 2017; Silverman et al., 2017).

Because of these negative reactions and responses, these simulations are generally not recommended. Instead, it is more effective to have students get to know people with disability who can share their experiences and give students more realistic and positive views of people with disability.

COMMUNICATION BARRIERS

Communication between healthcare professionals and their patients or clients is essential to the therapeutic relationship. Yet, communication barriers are among the most common types of barriers experienced by people with disability (as reported in studies by Smeltzer,

Avery, and Haynor [2012] and many others). Communication barriers might include the following:

- Talking to an accompanying person rather than the person with a disability

- Failing to provide people with disability the information about health issues they need and consider important

- Communicating with and treating people with disability as if they were children

- Failing to ask people with a disability what is the best way to communicate with them

- Failing to use alternative communication strategies for people with disability

- Pretending to understand what a person with disability has said

- Failing to include people with disability in discussions and decisions about their own care

- Failing to recognize that some people with disability have a low reading level or low health literacy

> Communication barriers affect all persons with disabilities, not only those with hearing, vision, and communication impairment.

Another communication barrier is the discomfort some healthcare professionals feel about asking patients about their disability and its effects on their health and everyday lives. This is often because healthcare professionals lack knowledge about disability, have had little previous contact with people with disability, or fear they will offend or upset patients with disability. Although asking a stranger such questions in a social setting would indeed be inappropriate and insensitive, doing so in a health-related interaction is appropriate. This is because the presence of a disability may have a direct impact on a patient's health as well as that patient's ability to participate in health-promotion activities, follow a treatment regimen, or undergo preventive screening. Indeed, *not* asking about the effects of a disability on a patient's life and activities may distress the patient because it suggests that the healthcare provider has not considered the disability and its possible effects on the patient's health. A simple approach is to say to the individual with a disability, "Please tell me about your disability." Patients with disability are often the most knowledgeable and most expert persons about their disability. They are usually able and eager to explain their health issues and to provide useful information to healthcare professionals. They just need to be asked.

One of the most challenging scenarios for healthcare providers involves interacting with patients who are nonverbal or whose speech is difficult to understand. This may occur with people with severe intellectual or developmental disabilities or adults with aphasia due to stroke or other neurological disorders. Speech and language therapists can often help healthcare providers (and individuals with disability and their family members) in this scenario by identifying or establishing alternate communication methods. In any case, it is critical that healthcare providers recognize that absence of verbal language does not mean that a patient is unable to hear or understand what is being said, so they should speak to these patients directly.

CONSEQUENCES OF COMMUNICATION BARRIERS

Communication barriers have several critical consequences. For example:

- They can lead to misinformation, an incomplete picture of the health status of the patient, unaddressed or unmet healthcare needs, errors, unsafe practices, and increased morbidity and mortality.

- Healthcare professionals who fail to use effective communication strategies with patients with disability can cause these individuals to feel angry, frustrated, or dissatisfied with their care, resulting in their reluctance or even refusal to seek care in the future.

- Healthcare professionals who fail to use alternative modes of communication with people who require accommodations because of a disability can compromise care.

- Asking family members or others accompanying the patient to provide information about a patient with disability or serve as interpreters without the patient's explicit permission is demeaning, violates the patient's privacy, and ignores the rights of people with disability to self-determination.

> Healthcare professionals must talk directly to patients with disability. Talking to accompanying persons rather than those with disability fails to acknowledge that those with disability are individuals who are capable and interested in the world around them.

STRATEGIES TO ADDRESS COMMUNICATION BARRIERS

Strategies for healthcare professionals and educators to address communication barriers include the following:

- Assuming that people with disability are capable of understanding and addressing their own needs

- Communicating with and treating adult patients with disability as such

- Recognizing that the presence of a disability, no matter how severe, does not mean that people with disability are unable to identify or communicate their needs

- Understanding that most people with disability are intelligent and knowledgeable about their health and disability and capable of making their own decisions about their care

- Speaking directly to people with disability rather than about them to family members or others who are accompanying them

- Referring to people with disability with person-first language (unless the person prefers otherwise)—for example, saying "person with a disability" rather than "disabled person" or "the disabled"

- Using the preferred method of communication for people with communication impairment

- If necessary, obtaining input from family members or other caregivers about the best way to communicate with a patient whose communication or cognition is impaired

Using person-first language emphasizes the person rather than the disability. When we think of the person first, we are more likely to see people with disability in a positive light and be more effective in our communication with them (Tennessee Disability Pathfinder, n.d.).

- Recognizing that some people with disability might not be able to decipher handwritten notes or instructions

- Using plain and simple wording to make information available to people with or without disabilities—for example, people with low literacy levels or whose first language is not English

- Not pretending to understand what people with impaired speech have said and instead asking them to repeat themselves or to use an alternative method of communication

- Learning and using accommodations for people with disability

- Asking people with disability their views on the topic being discussed

- Educating other healthcare providers about the disability-related competencies expected of them

- Using communication boards

Patients with some disabling conditions such as hearing loss, vision impairment, and cognitive impairment require special communication strategies. When interacting with a patient with hearing loss, the method of communication used will depend on the type and severity of the impairment. It is important to keep these points in mind:

> Some patients have more than one type of communication impairment. In this case, healthcare professionals must adjust communication efforts to meet the patient's needs, preferences, and abilities.

- As people age, they often develop hearing loss. Most of these people communicate with spoken language, which may be assisted with hearing aids.

- People with profound hearing loss that was present at birth or before they developed language skills will likely use sign language or speechreading. Communication must match the severity and type of hearing loss and the person's ability to communicate using alternate approaches.

- For many people who are Deaf (the uppercase "D" indicating hearing impairment from a very early age), sign language is their first language. This makes reading English more difficult for some.

Recommendations for communicating with people with hearing loss include the following:

- Use videos with closed captioning.

- Provide written materials.

- Provide audio-induction loops.

- Provide text telephones (TTY or TDD).

- For people whose first language is sign language, provide a sign-language interpreter or use pictures instead of words.

Like hearing impairment, vision loss varies in type and severity. When communicating with people with vision loss, it is important to consider the following points:

- When meeting a person with vision loss, announce your presence, address the person by name, and explain who you are, your role, what you will be doing, and what you will ask the individual to do.

- Speak directly to the person in a normal tone and volume. Do not shout and don't exaggerate or over-articulate when speaking.

- Do not rely on gestures (including head shakes or nods) to communicate with people with vision loss. They may be unable to see them.

- Use large-print documents for people with some vision loss.

- Provide or allow audio recordings of discussions. This enables the person to relisten to the discussion and to any instructions given.

- Offer Braille versions of written materials.

Effective communication with people with cognitive impairment can be challenging for many healthcare professionals, especially if they have little experience interacting with patients with cognitive issues. Cognitive impairment can occur in people with intellectual disability, developmental disability, head injury, neurological disorders, and dementia. Because some patients with intellectual disability may have difficulty communicating their needs, nursing staff must be especially attentive to them and perhaps use alternative communication strategies (e.g., the use of pictures) to provide quality nursing care (Ailey, Johnson, Fogg, & Friese, 2015).

Demonstrating patience is important when interacting with any patient, whether that patient has a disability or not. However, it is especially critical when communicating with patients with cognitive impairment.

Factors that determine the effectiveness of communication with people with cognitive disability include the following:

- The ability of the healthcare provider to establish trust

- Treating the person with dignity

- Communicating in a way that promotes comprehension at the person's level—for example, using short sentences and language the individual will understand

- Giving the person sufficient time to respond

- Using the person's name

- Treating persons with disability as adults even if their behavior or intellectual level is that of a child

For any person who has difficulty communicating, regardless of the reason why, a communication board can be an effective tool. A communication board is a device with a series of symbols, letters, words, and pictures from which persons with impaired communication can select to communicate with others. Speech-to-text and text-to-speech computer devices are also available to promote communication.

Additional strategies to communicate with individuals with hearing loss, vision loss, or cognitive impairment are discussed in more detail later in this book.

STRUCTURAL AND PHYSICAL BARRIERS

Structural and physical barriers in the built environment are perhaps the most visible and recognizable barriers. These include the following:

- Inaccessible parking areas

- The absence of ramps and curb cuts

- Steps outside buildings that hamper entry and steps inside buildings that prevent movement from floor to floor

- Narrow doorways that do not accommodate wheelchairs or other mobility devices
- Heavy doors or a lack of automatic doors
- Doorknobs that cannot be used by people with limited hand function
- Inadequate space
- The absence of height-adjustable examination tables, scales, and imaging equipment
- A lack of grab bars
- The absence of ramps or ramps that are too steep
- A lack of accessible restrooms
- Reception desks that are too high to permit people with disability to speak easily with receptionists
- Poor signage
- Forms (consent and otherwise) with small print or complex language
- A lack of knowledge about legal requirements for healthcare and other settings to accommodate people with disability

CONSEQUENCES OF STRUCTURAL AND PHYSICAL BARRIERS

The presence of structural and physical barriers limits access to both healthcare settings and healthcare in general—a major cause of poor healthcare among people with mobility limitations and similar types of disability.

STRATEGIES TO ADDRESS STRUCTURAL AND PHYSICAL BARRIERS

The Americans with Disabilities Act (ADA) requires that sites, settings, and facilities that are likely to be frequented by people with disability—for example, hospitals, clinics, private offices, imaging centers, clinical laboratories, urgent care centers, and so on—be accessible. Legal mandates also require that new construction and structures undergoing renovation be made accessible.

Even sites that are ADA compliant may still be inaccessible. To identify structural barriers to care, facilities must perform an accessibility assessment. Often, people with disability are the only ones able to provide an accurate assessment of a facility. Thus, they must be part of the assessment. The following sidebar offers additional information about accessibility assessment as well as on universal design, whose principles can be applied to increase accessibility for people with disability.

> The US government offers tax breaks to remove structural and physical barriers from facilities to enable people with disability to use health-related and other facilities

In addition to the accommodations mandated by the ADA, there are several low-cost strategies for reducing structural and physical barriers to care (especially for people who use wheelchairs):

- Moving chairs that obstruct pathways

- Removing deep-pile rugs or carpets

- Providing rooms with accessible tables and weight scales

- Using height-adjustable exam tables (some are expensive, but less costly options exist)

- Ensuring staff are available to help patients transfer to and from exam tables

- Modifying doors to easily swing both ways

- Installing grab bars in restroom stalls

- Placing hooks low on the back of restroom stall doors

SOURCES OF INFORMATION ON ACCESSIBILITY ASSESSMENT AND UNIVERSAL DESIGN

Multiple assessment guides exist. These can be used to ensure that sites are accessible. Following are links to useful resources for accessibility assessment:

- ADAAG Manual: A Guide to the Americans with Disabilities Act by the Access Board: https://www.adainfo.org/sites/default/files/ADAAG-Manual.pdf

- Survey Instruments to Assess Patient Experiences with Access Coordination Across Healthcare Settings: Available and Needed Measures by Quinn et al.: https://www.ncbi.nlm.nih.gov/pmc/articles/PMC5509356/

- Web Accessibility Evaluation Tools List by the Web Accessibility Initiative: https://www.w3.org/WAI/ER/tools/

For information about universal design, see the following resources:

- The 7 Principles by the National Disability Authority Centre for Excellence in Universal Design: http://universaldesign.ie/What-is-Universal-Design/The-7-Principles/

- Principles of Universal Design by the United States Access Board: https://www.access-board.gov/guidelines-and-standards/communications-and-it/26-255-guidelines/825-principles-of-universal-design

- The Seven Principles of Universal Design by Rosemarie Rossetti: https://www.udll.com/media-room/articles/the-seven-principles-of-universal-design/

Accessible sites and equipment also make life easier for certain people without disability—for example, people pushing children in strollers, people carrying groceries or making deliveries, older people, and people who are short in stature.

Healthcare professionals might consider elimination of physical and structural barriers to be beyond their expertise and outside their area of responsibility. But these barriers affect patient care, so addressing them is relevant to their role. In collaboration with people with disability, healthcare professionals are in a position to inform administrators when barriers exist and advocate for the adoption of strategies to minimize them.

Healthcare professionals must also understand and advocate for *reasonable accommodations*. This term refers to modifications made to tasks and to the environment to allow people with disability an equal opportunity to participate. This concept, often discussed in the context of employment and education, also applies in healthcare settings (Institute of Medicine, 2007).

To ensure that accessibility requirements are met, healthcare professionals must understand and educate others about accessibility.

PROGRAMMATIC BARRIERS

Examples of programmatic barriers in healthcare include the following:

- Inconvenient scheduling of healthcare visits

- Allowing too little time to accomplish needed assessments and healthcare interventions

- A lack of knowledge and expertise on the part of health-care providers about the health-related needs of people with disability

- A lack of training for healthcare staff to assist patients with disability so that both patients and healthcare personnel are safe

CONSEQUENCES OF PROGRAMMATIC BARRIERS

People with mobility limitations might need more time to travel to a healthcare facility—especially if they rely on paratransit services. (These are discussed in more detail in the later section

"Transportation Barriers.") They might also need more time and assistance during appointments to compensate for difficulties with undressing and transferring to the exam table. Scheduling appointments at inconvenient times (e.g., early in the day) and failing to allot adequate time to complete needed assessments and interventions increase stress on both patients and healthcare providers. Such scheduling issues can also result in patients missing important services (such as diagnostic tests or physical therapy sessions).

A lack of training and knowledge among staff as to how best to communicate with and to assist patients with disability may put these patients at risk of receiving misinformation and of experiencing falls or injuries. They can also increase risk of injury to staff.

STRATEGIES TO ADDRESS PROGRAMMATIC BARRIERS

Programmatic barriers are comparatively easy to address. Strategies include the following:

- Providing healthcare professionals with educational and training resources as well as teaching materials on disability (including information on the increased health risks associated with having a disability), caring for people with disability, and communication strategies

- Being aware of transportation barriers facing some patients with disability and scheduling them accordingly

- Scheduling multiple appointments for each visit to the healthcare setting to minimize the need for multiple trips

- Having alternative formats of materials available (e.g., large print, Braille, audio, consistent with patients' cognitive abilities)

PROVIDING QUALITY CARE FOR HOSPITALIZED PATIENTS WITH DISABILITY

People with disability who have been hospitalized have reported poor communication on the part of nursing staff and other healthcare providers, a lack of competence, compromised care, negative attitudes among staff, and a feeling of vulnerability (Smeltzer et al., 2012). Things are even worse for hospitalized patients with intellectual disability, who are at higher risk than other patients for complications (many of which are preventable) and require careful monitoring.

Patients with disability who require hospitalization need nurses and other healthcare providers to be knowledgeable about how to provide quality care. However, most healthcare professionals currently in practice have received little education about disability and have had limited opportunity to interact with patients with disability. Instruction and training can help with this. It can also allay providers' concerns and fears about working with patients with disability, uncover and dispel any implicit biases they may have, and learn techniques to ensure their safety as well as that of the patient. Finally, it can help them identify useful communication strategies for interacting with patients with disability. (Refer to the earlier section "Strategies to Address Communication Barriers" for more information.)

TRANSPORTATION BARRIERS

Multiple studies cite a lack of reliable and accessible transportation as one of the most common barriers to healthcare identified by people with disability. Despite an increase in the availability of public transportation since the passage of the ADA, transportation systems often fail to meet the needs of people with disability.

There are various reasons for this, including limited number of stops, inaccessible stations, and drivers who lack knowledge or harbor negative attitudes toward people with disability. In addition, *paratransit systems*—which are public transportation services designed for people with mobility limitations—are notoriously unreliable, arriving late or not at all (Bezyak, Sabella, & Gattis, 2017).

These problems have a disproportionate effect on people who are blind or have low vision and people who have mobility issues—particularly those who use wheelchairs. People who live in rural areas are at an even greater disadvantage due to a lack of public transportation options (National Council on Disability, 2015).

CONSEQUENCES OF TRANSPORTATION BARRIERS

People with disability who rely on paratransit systems are at risk for missed appointments, long wait times, missed pickups at the end of the day, and lengthy travel times. This causes many patients to give up on trying to obtain healthcare. As a result, health problems may be missed, or they may be diagnosed and treated late in their course. As a result, their health status and quality of life may suffer.

STRATEGIES TO ADDRESS TRANSPORTATION BARRIERS

Nurses and other healthcare professionals cannot remove transportation barriers. However, they can recognize these barriers and consider the difficulties they cause patients with disability who must depend on others for transportation in scheduling health-related appointments. Healthcare providers can also advocate for improved and more reliable transportation services for these patients, identify and recommend the use of more reliable accessible van services, and push for policy changes to address these barriers.

PUTTING IT ALL TOGETHER

Table 3.1 summarizes major categories of barriers, examples, and corrective practices to minimize them.

DISABILITY-RELATED COMPETENCIES FOR HEALTHCARE PROFESSIONS AND PROVIDERS

In an effort to ensure that healthcare professionals—including nurses, physicians, occupational and physical therapists, speech pathologists and therapists, and others involved in patient care—are adequately prepared to provide high-quality care to individuals with disability, several organizations have developed specific competencies. Several of these sets of competencies are described briefly here:

- **Alliance for Disability in Health Care Education, Inc. (ADHCE):** This organization, whose goal is the integration of disability-related content and concepts into the healthcare professions, developed *Core Competencies on Disability for Health Care Education*. The competencies are not discipline specific and are intended to be applicable to all healthcare professions and to all categories of clinicians (Alliance for Disability in Health Care Education, 2019).

- **American Nurses Association (ANA):** The ANA develops and publishes the scope and standards of practice related to intellectual and developmental disabilities nursing (American Nurses Association, 2013).

- **American Rehabilitation Counseling Association (ARCA):** The ARCA Task Force on Competencies for Counseling Persons with Disabilities has put forth a set of competencies for counselors who work with persons with disability in school, employment, community, and clinical settings (Chapin et al., 2018).

TABLE 3.1   BARRIERS TO HEALTHCARE ACCESS FOR PEOPLE WITH

CATEGORY	EXAMPLES
Attitudinal barriers	Negative attitudes among healthcare professionals toward people with disability, resulting in stereotyping, bias, stigma, prejudice, and discrimination
	A lack of knowledge about the abilities and strengths of people with disability
	The assumption that people with disability are dependent, unaware of or uninterested in events around them, and unable to make decisions or otherwise participate in life activities
	The belief that all health issues that affect people with disability are due to their disability (diagnostic overshadowing)
	The failure to recognize, prevent, and treat common health issues that affect those with and without disabilities
	The assumption that the quality of life of people with disability is poor
Communication barriers	Talking to an accompanying person rather than person with a disability
	Treating and communicating with people with disability as if they were children
	Failing to ask people with disability the best way to communicate with them
	Failing to use alternative communication strategies for people with disability
	Pretending you understand what a person with disability has said even if you do not
	Failing to include people with disability in discussions or decisions about their own care
	Failing to recognize people with disability with a low reading level or low health literacy
	Feeling uncomfortable asking patients about their disability and its effects on their general health for fear of offending the patient
	Failing to provide people with disability the information about their health issues they need and consider important

DISABILITY, EXAMPLES, AND CORRECTIVE PRACTICES

CORRECTIVE PRACTICES

Educate people without knowledge or exposure to people with disability.

Provide experiences with people with varied disabilities to increase knowledge and comfort level.

Model positive behaviors when interacting with people with disability.

Educate others about the need for people with disability to receive the same quality of care, including health promotion and preventive screening, as that provided to others.

Do not ignore others' negative behaviors toward people with disability.

Include standardized patients with disability in health professions education.

Include people with disability on the education team.

Learn and use accommodations for people with disability.

Obtain input from family caregivers about the best way to communicate with people with communication or cognitive impairment.

Ask people with disability their views on the topic being discussed

View people with disability as the decision-makers for their own care.

Involve people with disability in decision-making about their health and well-being.

Educate other healthcare providers about the disability-related competencies expected of them.

Use person-first language when referring to people with disability.

Increase own knowledge about health issues of those with disability.

Assume people with disability can understand and address their own needs.

Treat and communicate with adult patients as such.

Recognize that the presence of a disability does not mean people are unable to identify or communicate their own needs, and that most people with disability are intelligent and knowledgeable about their own health and disability.

Speak directly to people with disability rather than about them to those accompanying them.

Understand that some people with disability might not be able to decipher handwritten notes or instructions.

Use plain and simple wording.

continues

TABLE 3.1   BARRIERS TO HEALTHCARE ACCESS FOR PEOPLE WITH

CATEGORY	EXAMPLES
Communi-cation barriers (continued)	

DISABILITY, EXAMPLES, AND CORRECTIVE PRACTICES (CONT.)

CORRECTIVE PRACTICES

Do not pretend to understand what people with impaired speech have said. Instead, ask them to repeat themselves or use an alternative method of communication.

Use a communication board, text-to-speech, and speech-to-text devices.

For people with hearing impairment:

Use videos with closed captioning.

Provide written materials.

Provide audio-induction loops.

Provide text telephones (TTY or TDD).

For people whose first language is sign language, provide a sign-language interpreter or use pictures instead of words.

For people with vision impairment:

Use large print in documents.

Use audio recordings.

Offer Braille versions of written materials.

Employ tools available on smartphones and other technological devices.

When meeting a patient with vision loss, announce your presence, address the patient by name, and explain who you are, what your role is, what you will be doing, and what you will ask the patient to do.

Speak directly to the patient in a normal tone and volume. Do not shout.

Do not rely on gestures (including head shakes or nods) to communicate with people with vision loss. They may be unable to see them.

For people with cognitive impairment:

Use reading and language levels appropriate for the individual.

Use pictures instead of words.

Establish trust.

Treat patients with dignity.

Communicate in a way that promotes comprehension at the patient's level—for example, using short sentences and language the individual will understand.

Give patients sufficient time to respond.

Use the patient's name.

Treat patients as adults even if their behavior or intellectual level is that of a child.

continues

TABLE 3.1 BARRIERS TO HEALTHCARE ACCESS FOR PEOPLE WITH

CATEGORY	EXAMPLES
Structural and physical barriers	Inaccessible parking areas
	The absence of ramps and curb cuts
	Steps outside buildings that hamper entry and steps inside buildings that prevent movement from floor to floor
	Narrow doorways that do not accommodate wheelchairs or other mobility devices
	Heavy doors or a lack of automatic doors or door openers
	Doorknobs that cannot be used by people with limited hand function
	The absence of height-adjustable examination tables, scales, and imaging equipment
	A lack of grab bars
	A lack of accessible restrooms
	Poor signage
	A lack of knowledge about legal requirements for healthcare and other settings to accommodate people with disability
	Inadequate space
	The absence of ramps or ramps that are too steep
	Reception desks that are too high to permit people with disability to speak easily with receptionists
	Forms (consent and otherwise) with small print or complex language
Program-matic barriers	Inconvenient scheduling of healthcare visits
	Allowing too little time to accomplish needed assessments and healthcare interventions
	A lack of knowledge and expertise on the part of healthcare providers about the health-related needs of people with disability
	A lack of training of healthcare staff to assist patients with disability so that both patients and healthcare personnel are safe
Transporta-tion barriers	Lack of accessible public transportation
	Unreliable transportation

(CDC, n.d.-a; -b)

DISABILITY, EXAMPLES, AND CORRECTIVE PRACTICES (CONT.)

CORRECTIVE PRACTICES

Advocate for accessible entrances into and within buildings used by the public.

Ask a person with disability to evaluate sites for accessibility.

Inform administrators of a lack of accessible site and equipment.

Become knowledgeable about laws that address the legal rights of people with disability to accommodations and accessible facilities.

Educate and advocate for greater understanding of legal requirements to make reasonable accommodations for people with disability.

If the accessibility of a site or setting is questionable, use an accessibility form to evaluate it.

Move chairs that obstruct pathways.

Remove deep-pile rugs or carpets.

Provide rooms with accessible tables and weight scales.

Use height-adjustable exam tables. (Some are expensive, but less costly options exist.)

Ensure staff are available to help patients transfer to and from exam tables.

Modify doors to easily swing both ways.

Install grab bars in restroom stalls.

Place hooks low on the back of restroom stall doors.

Provide educational and training resources as well as teaching materials about caring for people with disability to all providers across the healthcare continuum.

Modify scheduling to allow for adequate time and assistance (if needed) to ensure high-quality care for people with disability.

Train staff to assist and transfer patients in a way that is safe for both patients and staff.

Offer alternative formats of materials (large print, Braille, audio) consistent with patients' cognitive abilities.

Educate healthcare professionals about the increased health risks associated with having a disability.

Advocate for accessible transportation systems.

Identify and recommend use of *reliable* accessible van services.

Push for policy changes to address transportation barriers.

- **Council on Social Work Education (CSWE):** The CSWE's Council on Disability and Persons with Disability has developed competencies for disability-competent care and identified resources to support the inclusion of disability-related content and concepts in social work education. The resources could be useful for other disciplines interested in ensuring the preparation of health professions students to care for individuals with disability (Council on Social Work Education Disability Competent Care Curriculum Workshop, 2018).

- **Developmental Disabilities Nurses Association (DDNA):** This organization has developed practice standards to promote quality nursing care of people with developmental disabilities. The organization provides support to nurses who specialize in caring for individuals with developmental disabilities.

Although several of these sets of standards and competencies were developed to be specific to one profession or another, much could be gained by examining how various healthcare disciplines address the health issues and care of individuals with disability. This is particularly important because of the interprofessional collaboration that is needed to ensure a high level of healthcare to individuals with disability. Several of these sets of competencies also identify resources to promote the integration of disability-specific content in educational curricula. These resources could be useful for any discipline or healthcare professional interested in disability.

SUMMARY

This chapter has discussed in detail barriers facing many people with disability. Some of these barriers make it difficult for people with disability to obtain quality healthcare; others make it impossible. Implicit bias has been identified as an underlying factor in attitudinal barriers that result in negative attitudes toward people with disability. This bias also prevents healthcare professionals from recognizing the stereotyping, prejudice, and discriminatory practices that affect the quality of care provided to this population. Another major factor underlying the barriers addressed here is inadequate attention to disability and its impact on health and healthcare in the educational preparation of healthcare professionals. This chapter identified strategies to address the various barriers to healthcare; they will be discussed further in subsequent chapters that address specific categories of disabilities.

REFERENCES

Ailey, S. H., Johnson, T. J., Fogg, L., & Friese, T. R. (2015). Factors related to complications among adult patients with intellectual disabilities hospitalized at an academic medical center. *Intellectual and Developmental Disabilities, 53*(2), 114–119. doi: 10.1352/1934-9556-53.2.114

Alliance for Disability in Health Care Education. (2019). Core competencies on disability for health care education. Retrieved from http://www.adhce.org/resources/core-competencies-on-disability-for-health-care-education/

American Bar Association Commission on Disability Rights. (2019). Implicit biases & people with disabilities. Retrieved from https://www.americanbar.org/groups/diversity/disabilityrights/resources/implicit_bias

American Nurses Association. (2013). *Intellectual and developmental disabilities nursing: Scope and standards of practice.* Washington, DC: ANA.

Bersani, H., & Lyman, L. M. (2009). Governmental policies and programs for people with disabilities. In C. E. Drum, G. L. Krahn, & H. Bersani (Eds), *Disability and public health* (pp. 79–104). Washington, D.C.: American Public Health Association.

Bezyak, J. L., Sabella, S. A., & Gattis, R. H. (2017). Public transportation: An investigation of barriers for people with disabilities. *Journal of Disability Policy Studies, 28(1),* 52–60. doi:10.1177/1044207317702070

Centers for Disease Control and Prevention. (n.d.-a). Common barriers to participation experienced by people with disabilities. Retrieved from https://www.cdc.gov/ncbddd/disabilityandhealth/disability-barriers.html

Centers for Disease Control and Prevention. (n.d.-b). Disability and health inclusion strategies. Retrieved from https://www.cdc.gov/ncbddd/disabilityandhealth/disability-strategies.html

Chapin, M., McCarthy, H., Shaw, L., Bradham-Cousar, M., Chapman, R., Nosek, M., ... Ysasi, N. (2018). Disability-related counseling competencies. Alexandria, VA: American Rehabilitation Counseling Association.

Council on Social Work Education. Disability-Competent Care Curriculum Workgroup. (2018). Curricular resource on issues of disability and disability-competent care. Retrieved from https://cswe.org/Centers-Initiatives/Centers/Center-for-Diversity/Curricular-Resource-on-Issues-of-Disability-and-Di.aspx

Institute of Medicine. (2007). *The future of disability in America.* Washington, D.C.: The National Academies Press.

Long-Bellil, L. M., Robey, K. L., Graham, C. L., Minihan, P. M., Smeltzer, S. C, & Kahn, P. (2011). Teaching medical students about disability: The use of standardized patients. *Academic Medicine, 86*(9), 1,163–1,170. doi:10.1097/ACM.0b013e318226b5dc

Nario-Redmond, M. R., Gospodinov, D., & Cobb, A. (2017). Crip for a day: The unintended negative consequences of disability simulations. *Rehabilitation Psychology, 62*(3), 324–333. doi:10.1037/rep0000127

National Council on Disability. (2015). Transportation update: Where we've gone and what we've learned. Retrieved from https://ncd.gov/publications/2015/05042015/

Pelleboer-Gunnink, H. A., Van Oorsouw, W. M. W. J., Van Weeghel, J., & Embregts, P. J. C. M. (2017). Mainstream health professionals' stigmatising attitudes towards people with intellectual disabilities: A systematic review. *Journal of Intellectual Disability Research, 61*(5), 411–434. doi:10.1111/jir.12353

Shakespeare, T., & Kleine, I. (2013). Educating health professionals about disability: A review of interventions. *Health and Social Care Education, 2*(2), 20–37.

Silverman, A. M., Pitonyak, J. S., Nelson, I. K., Matsuda, P. N., Kartin, D., & Molton, I. R. (2017). Instilling positive beliefs about disabilities: Pilot testing a novel experiential learning activity for rehabilitation students. *Disability and Rehabilitation, 40*(9), 1,108–1,113. doi:10.1080/09638288.2017.1292321

Smeltzer, S. C., Avery, C., & Haynor, P. (2012). Interactions of people with disabilities with nursing staff during hospitalization. *American Journal of Nursing, 112*(4), 30–37. doi:10.1097/01.NAJ.0000413454.07369.e3

Smeltzer, S. C., Ross, J. G., Mariani, B., Meakim, C. H., Bruderle, E., de Mange, E., & Nthenge, S. (2018). Innovative approach to address disability concepts and standardized patients with disability in an undergraduate curriculum. *Journal of Nursing Education, 57*(12), 760–764. doi:10.3928/01484834-20181119-11

Symons, A. B., Morley, C. P., McGuigan, D., & Akl, E. A. (2014). A curriculum on care for people with disabilities: Effects on medical student self-reported attitudes and comfort level. *Disability and Health Journal, 7*(1), 88–95. doi: 10.1016/j.dhjo.2013.08.006

Tennessee Disability Pathfinder. (n.d.) Disability Etiquette & People First Language. Retrieved from https://cme.mc.vanderbilt.edu/sites/default/files/TennesseeDisabilityPathfinder-DisabilityEtiquettePeopleFirstLanguage%2812811%29.pdf

Tervo, R. C., Palmer, G., & Redinius, P. (2004). Health professional student attitudes towards people with disability. *Clinical rehabilitation, 18*(8), 908–915. https://doi.org/10.1191/0269215504cr820oa

VanPuymbrouck, L., Heffron, J. L., Sheth, A. J., The, K. J., & Lee, D. (2017). Experiential learning: Critical analysis of standardized patient and disability simulation. *Journal of Occupational Therapy Education, 1*(3). doi:10.26681/jote.2017.010305

Vest, B. M., Lynch, A., McGuigan, D., Servoss, T., Zinnerstrom, K., & Symons, A. B. (2016). Using standardized patient encounters to teach longitudinal continuity of care in a family medicine clerkship. *BMC Medical Education, 16*(1), 208. doi:10.1186/s12909-016-0733-y

Woodard, L. J., Havercamp, S. M., Zwygart, K. K., & Perkins, E. A. (2012). An innovative clerkship module focused on patients with disabilities. *Academic Medicine, 87*(4), 537–542. doi:10.1097/ACM.0b013e318248ed0a

World Health Organization. (2011). World report on disability. Retrieved from https://www.who.int/publications/i/item/world-report-on-disability

---

4

INTELLECTUAL AND DEVELOPMENTAL DISABILITIES

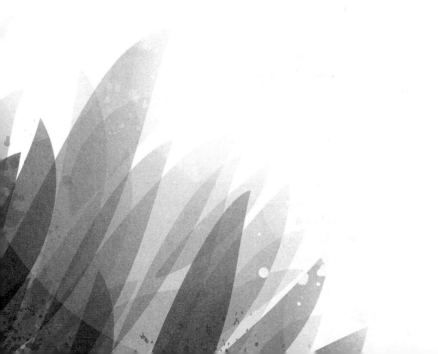

INTRODUCTION

Developmental disability is an umbrella term that includes several types of lifelong and often severe disabilities that occur before the age of 22. Some developmental disabilities are largely physical in nature, such as osteogenesis imperfecta, cerebral palsy, and dwarfism. Others involve both physical and intellectual disability, such as Down syndrome and fetal alcohol syndrome. Others are intellectual disorders, such as autism spectrum disorder. Developmental disabilities that affect cognitive function are identified as intellectual disability (Centers for Disease Control and Prevention [CDC], n.d.-h; Schalock et al., 2012).

Intellectual disability is not a single disorder. Rather, the term is used to describe general symptoms of neurologic dysfunction (Shea, 2012). An intellectual disability is a developmental disability that occurs before the age of 18 and involves impaired intellectual functioning, a limited ability to function in daily life, and an impaired ability to learn, reason, and problem-solve. Additionally, intellectual disability is characterized by limited adaptive behavior, including a range of everyday social and practical skills (CDC, n.d.-e; Schalock et al., 2012).

> Definitions of intellectual and developmental disabilities (IDDs) differ somewhat from one source to the other.

Intellectual disability is broadly related to thought processes and is characterized by significant limitations in intellectual functioning and adaptive behavior. These can be categorized as follows (Schalock et al., 2012):

- **Conceptual skills:** These are the language and literacy skills used to manage money and time, understand number concepts, and be self-directive.

- **Social skills:** These include interpersonal skills and self-esteem, as well as an understanding of concepts like social responsibility and social problem-solving; the ability to follow rules, obey laws, and avoid being victimized; and a lack of gullibility and naïveté (in other words, a healthy sense of wariness).

- **Practical skills:** These include skills needed to carry out activities of daily living (personal care), occupational skills, skills to access healthcare, skills to travel or use transportation, the ability to maintain schedules and routines, money skills, the ability to use the telephone, and safety skills.

By definition, intellectual disability occurs any time before the age of 18. However, it is often diagnosed or observed soon after birth or during early childhood—although it is not diagnosed in some children until they are in school. Children with intellectual disability tend to have difficulty learning to speak, walk, dress, and eat without assistance, and have difficulty learning in school. Children with intellectual disability may be slower or fail in achieving developmental milestones expected of children (CDC, n.d.-b). Children and adults with intellectual disability often have difficulty letting others know their needs and wants, and many are unable to take care of themselves.

Although these disabilities are lifelong, functioning of many people with intellectual disability can be enhanced through appropriate supports, including early interventions (Schalock et al., 2012). There are varying degrees of intellectual disability, from mild to profound. Many people with intellectual disability can and do learn new skills. However, they often learn them more slowly, and usually only with support from others. With others' support, many are able to be successful at school and work and to establish relationships with others.

Many people with intellectual disability have also been successful in advocating for themselves and for others with disability. As self-advocates, they exercise their decision-making role related to aspects of their daily lives, including their health and healthcare. Many people with IDD live full lives in their community, live independently or with their families, have rewarding jobs, and contribute to society. Further, they exercise their rights in public policy that affects them and others with IDD, which is consistent with the principle, "Nothing about me without me" (The ARC, 2014).

OTHER TERMINOLOGY

The term *mental retardation*, once used to describe intellectual disability, has been removed from the international classification systems of diseases and disabilities, agencies and professional organizations, names of national committees, and journal titles (Harris, 2013; Schalock et al., 2012; Social Security Administration, 2013). Adopting the term *intellectual disability* in its place eliminates the use of the former pejorative or negative term and emphasizes that intervention is warranted early in the developmental period. Other terms used in place of mental retardation are intellectual developmental disorders, developmental delay, general learning disability, and neurodevelopmental disorder.

The euphemism *special needs*, as in special-needs children, is frequently used to soften the image of a person with disability. However, many disability advocates and organizations caution against the use of this term for several reasons:

- "Special needs" is not a legal term.
- It is imprecise and not meaningful.
- It is seen as offensive by many disability advocates because it stigmatizes persons with disability by avoiding correct terminology.
- It is seen as patronizing and condescending.

A recent study revealed that the term *special needs* was viewed more negatively by the population at large than the use of the more accurate term *disability* (Gernsbacher, Raimond, Balinghasay, & Boston, 2016). Despite recommendations against use of this term, however, it is one that nurses, nursing students, and other healthcare providers will encounter. Other terms, such as physically challenged or differently abled, are also euphemisms that should be avoided. It is recommended that correct terminology be used instead. It is important, however, to be guided by what terms people with disability prefer (or, in the case of children, what their parents prefer). As described in Chapter 2, person-first language is preferable in any circumstance.

PREVALENCE OF INTELLECTUAL AND DEVELOPMENTAL DISABILITY

In 2017, about 1 in 6 children ages 3 to 17 were reported by their parents as having been diagnosed with developmental disability (Zablotsky et al., 2019). This translates to 17.8% of children 3 to 17 years of age—an increase from 16.2% in 2009. Increases have also been reported in the prevalence of attention-deficit/hyperactivity disorder, autism spectrum disorder (ASD), and intellectual disability, with a significant decrease for other developmental delays. The prevalence of developmental disability increased among boys, older children, Hispanic children, and non-Hispanic white children. These increases have been attributed in part to improved awareness and better screening, diagnoses, and access to services (CDC, n.d.-h). In a study of 8-year-olds in metropolitan Atlanta, Braun et al. (2015) reported no differences in prevalence of intellectual disability, cerebral palsy, or hearing impairment from 1993 to 2010, but a slight increase in vision impairment and a significant increase in the prevalence of ASD. (ASD is discussed later in this chapter.)

Using data from the U.S. Census Bureau, Larson et al. (2018) estimated the number of people in the US with IDD to be more than 7.3 million, or 22.8 per 1,000 people in 2016. Of these, more than 5 million were children and almost 2 million were adults in the civilian noninstitutionalized US population. Another estimate indicates that between 2.5 and 4 million adults in the US have an intellectual disability (Lauer & McCallion, 2015) and an even larger population has developmental disability. These differences in estimates are due in part to different sources of data and different definitions of intellectual and developmental disability. In addition, many individuals with IDD and other types of disability have not been included in national surveys and registries.

The international prevalence of intellectual disability is about 1%, depending on socioeconomic status and other factors that vary across countries (McKenzie, Milton, Smith, & Ouellette-Kuntz, 2016).

CAUSES OF INTELLECTUAL AND DEVELOPMENTAL DISABILITY

IDD is caused by numerous and complex factors (CDC, n.d.-h). These factors include but are not limited to the following:

- Genetics

- Parental health and behaviors (e.g., smoking and alcohol consumption)

- Exposure of the mother to environmental toxins during pregnancy

- Injury or perinatal asphyxia at the time of delivery

Fetal alcohol syndrome, genetic and chromosomal conditions (such as Down syndrome and fragile X syndrome), and certain infections during pregnancy are known causes of intellectual disability. Other factors associated with increased risk of intellectual disability include the following:

- Low birth weight

- Premature birth

- Multiple birth

Preventable causes of intellectual disability include malnutrition and iodine deficiency in the mother during pregnancy and malnutrition of the mother or child (Chiurazzi & Pirozzi, 2016). A rare cause of these disabilities is elevated bilirubin level in a newborn's blood. If untreated, this can cause brain damage resulting in a variety of disorders, including cerebral palsy and hearing, vision, and intellectual impairment. Intellectual disability can also occur as part of other disorders that affect other body systems (Chiurazzi & Pirozzi, 2016).

Despite these known causes, the factors that cause intellectual and developmental disability often cannot be determined. Although genetic defects such as chromosomal abnormalities may cause disability, these are not inherited. Down syndrome, which is the most common genetic cause of intellectual disability, is an example of a noninherited genetic abnormality or mutation.

Even if an intellectual or developmental disability is not obvious in a newborn and may not become evident until a child begins school, many of these disabilities begin before birth or with injury, infection, or other factors at the time of birth. Intellectual and developmental disability can occur at any time during the developmental years and usually lasts throughout a person's lifetime (CDC, n.d.-h).

> More than 800 genes are known to be involved in conditions associated with intellectual disability (Chiurazzi & Pirozzi, 2016).

CONSEQUENCES OF INTELLECTUAL AND DEVELOPMENTAL DISABILITY

Intellectual and developmental disability can result in several secondary conditions. A *secondary condition* is one that occurs or is more likely to occur because of the presence of a disability. Many secondary conditions are predictable and preventable. These include the following:

- Bowel or bladder problems
- Fatigue
- Injury
- Depression and other mental health problems
- Overweight and obesity
- Pain
- Pressure ulcers
- Poor oral and dental health
- Osteoporosis

People with IDD are also more likely than those without disability to experience higher rates of the following (Traci, Seekins, Szalda-Petree, & Ravesloot, 2002):

- Epilepsy
- Psychiatric disorders
- Gastrointestinal disorders
- Sensory impairment
- Limited mobility

Overweight and obesity are more common in youth with IDD than their nondisabled peers and are accompanied by increased prevalence of high blood cholesterol levels, preoccupation with weight, diabetes, and hypertension (Rimmer et al., 2010; WHO, 2011, 2018).

Chronic health conditions that may occur with IDD, depending on the specific type of IDD and its severity, include aspiration, dehydration, constipation, seizures, muscle spasm and contractures, gastroesophageal reflux, sleep disturbances, vision and hearing impairments, and others. The occurrence of these health conditions increases the complexity of care for those with IDD (Auberry, 2018).

In addition, this population is at increased risk for polypharmacy and the consequences of the use of multiple medications. It is also at risk for early mortality because of multiple health conditions and lack of adequate general healthcare (Lauer & McCallion, 2015). People with IDD often experience poor health and earlier onset of age-related conditions compared to their non-disabled peers—not only because of their disability, but because of a lack of attention to common preventable health issues. There is a reluctance or failure of many healthcare professionals to address health promotion and preventive care with people with IDD. This is in part because they believe that people with IDD:

- Are not interested in health promotion and disease prevention
- Are incapable of participating in such activities
- Will gain nothing because they already have disability

However, there is strong evidence that health promotion, including physical activity and exercise, can be effective in improving the health and the quality of life of people with IDD and other types of disability (US Department of Health and Human Services, 2018). Attention to oral and dental health is another important component of health promotion for people with IDD (National Institute of Dental and Craniofacial Research, n.d.; Fisher, 2004).

In addition to being at risk for secondary conditions related to IDD, people with these disabilities are at risk for the same health issues that affect people without disabilities, such as:

- Cardiovascular disease

- Diabetes

- Respiratory disease

- Cancer

In addition, they may be at higher risk than those without disability for certain disorders and health issues. Further, there is a risk of *diagnostic overshadowing*—that is, the tendency for healthcare providers to erroneously attribute all health issues to the person's disability. Thus, because healthcare providers often fail to address or even consider health promotion and disease prevention when caring for people with disability, they are also at risk for the following:

- Obesity

- Poor nutrition

- Lack of physical activity and exercise

- The effects of smoking

- Low bone density

It's true that people without disability fail to meet the recommendations for physical activity. However, the presence of an intellectual disability has been reported to be associated with even lower levels of physical activity among children and young adults; this increases their risk for chronic disease associated with a sedentary lifestyle

(Stanish, Curtin, Must, Phillips, Maslin, & Bandini, 2019). Health promotion programs with the goal of increased physical activity and improved nutritional status have been shown to be effective for those with IDD, including programs in which individuals with IDD served as cotrainers (Marks, Sisirak, Magallanes, Krok, & Donohue-Chase, 2019).

People with disability are at higher risk for abuse, including sexual abuse and assault. This risk is even higher for those with intellectual and developmental disability and those with psychiatric/mental health impairment. Children with mental or intellectual impairments are 4.6 times more likely to experience sexual violence than their nondisabled peers (Hughes et al., 2012).

Although life expectancy for people with IDD has increased in recent years, it remains lower than life expectancy for those without these disabilities. Moreover, mortality rates are higher for people with IDD (Lauer & McCallion, 2015). In the US, the average life expectancy of older adults with intellectual disability is currently 66.1 years. Although this is shorter than the 76.9 years of older adults without disability, it is considerably higher than a few years ago—and higher than what many healthcare professionals realize. For example, the life expectancy of people with Down syndrome is currently 60 years—up from 25 years in 1983 and 49 years in 1997 (CDC, n.d.-d; Fisher, 2012).

Because of their increased life expectancy, people with IDD and other disabilities are at risk for health issues that occur with aging such as bone loss and osteoporosis—often with an early onset—due in part to medications used to treat seizure disorders. An increased life expectancy for people with IDD also means they may outlive their parents and other caregivers, resulting in stress and fear on the part of parents and other family members about who will provide care for their children as they age. It is important to consider how disruptive a major change in living arrangements and availability of support can be to someone with an intellectual disability. The impact of such a change is even greater if the change in living arrangements and support is sudden and unexpected (Hahn et al., 2016).

Other transitions occur across the lifespan, including from childhood to adolescence to adulthood and older age, alterations in health status or function, changes in the immediate environment or living arrangement, changes in or loss of previous relationships and supports, and changes from pediatric to adult healthcare. It is important to anticipate transitions when possible and to engage the person with IDD, the person's family and support persons, and the interprofessional healthcare team to work together to minimize the stress and disruption that will occur with these transitions (Sullivan et al., 2011).

Nurses and other healthcare professionals can help people with IDD and their family caregiver or guardian prepare for changes and transitions that may occur and link them to resources that may be helpful in planning.

Another important issue is the increased incidence of psychiatric/mental health disorders in people with intellectual disability. The coexistence of intellectual disability and psychiatric/mental health illness is referred to as dual diagnosis. In the past, people with disability were not thought to have mental illnesses and were not evaluated or treated. While psychiatric/mental health disorders affect about 19% of the general population in the US, their prevalence in individuals with intellectual disability has been estimated to be more than 40% (Werner & Stawski, 2012). The impact of this dual diagnosis on the affected individuals, their family and caregivers, and support providers is considerable. Depression is common.

Psychiatric symptoms can include hyperactivity, self-injurious harmful behaviors (e.g., biting or beating one's head against a hard surface), and repetitive stereotyped behaviors. Healthcare professionals have been found to have low levels of knowledge or awareness of dual diagnosis, negative attitudes toward those with dual diagnosis, and overreliance on psychoactive medications rather than other treatment options, such as behavioral therapy. The use of psychotropic medications (e.g., antipsychotic agents, antidepressants, mood stabilizing agents), if not monitored appropriately, increases the risk of complications related to polypharmacy and drug interactions (Trollor, Salomon, & Franklin, 2016; Betz & Nehring, 2010).

Additionally, reliance on psychotropic medications alone to treat those with dual diagnosis or in response to disruptive behaviors can result in a lost opportunity for those with intellectual disability to receive and benefit from other therapy, such as behavioral or cognitive therapy (Ailey & Melich-Munyan, 2010).

It is also important to consider that challenging behaviors exhibited by persons with intellectual disability (e.g., outbursts of anger, irritability, aggression) may indicate the presence of pain, other discomfort, stress, an overly stimulating environment, or frustration because of their inability to communicate needs rather than a psychiatric/mental health issue. It is important to consider strategies to assess for and alleviate other causes of these behaviors rather than concluding prematurely that the behaviors indicate psychiatric/mental health disorders (Sullivan et al., 2011).

CHARACTERISTICS OF SELECT INTELLECTUAL AND DEVELOPMENTAL DISABILITIES

Some intellectual and developmental disabilities can be severe, with major effects on all aspects of a person's life. Others are less severe. Indeed, some types of mild intellectual or developmental disabilities could almost be an "invisible disability." That is, others might not know an individual had a disability unless that person shared that information.

The severity of a disability is linked to some extent to the cause, although the cause is often unknown, and to other accompanying disorders. For example, people with intellectual disability often have other disorders such as attention-deficit/hyperactivity disorder and autism spectrum disorder (Chiurazzi & Pirozzi, 2016). The specific features or characteristics of IDD depend on the disability and the type and severity of limitations. Table 4.1 identifies

The specific manifestations of an IDD that affect an individual dictate how to address specific issues when caring for that person and describes several common developmental disabilities (although the table is clearly limited in the number of disabilities included).

TABLE 4.1   DESCRIPTIONS AND CHARACTERISTICS OF SELECT INTELLECTUAL AND DEVELOPMENTAL DISABILITIES

GENERAL DESCRIPTION	COMMON FEATURES OR CHARACTERISTICS
ATTENTION-DEFICIT/HYPERACTIVITY DISORDER (ADHD)	
A neurobehavioral condition that interferes with a person's ability to pay attention and exercise age-appropriate inhibition. There are three types of ADHD: • Predominantly hyperactive-impulsive type (without significant inattention) • Predominantly inattentive type (without significant hyperactive-impulsive behavior) • Combination type (includes combination of hyperactive-impulsive and inattentive types) Combination type is the most common of the three types. 9.4% of children ages 2 to 17 and 4.4% of adults have been diagnosed with ADHD. The prevalence of ADHD is higher in males than females.	• Inattention (does not seem to listen) • Hyperactivity and impulsivity • Avoidance of activities requiring sustained mental effort • Difficulty organizing tasks and activities • Failure to complete activities or projects • Loses needed items • Forgetful of daily activities • Restlessness, fidgeting, or squirming (inability to sit still) • Has difficulty waiting in line or taking turns
AUTISM SPECTRUM DISORDER (ASD)	
A bio-neurological developmental disability that generally appears before the age of 3 and can cause significant social, communication, and behavioral challenges. ASD affects 1 in 59 children and 2.21% of adults (over 5 million adults in the US).	• Difficulty communicating and interacting with other people (may be nonverbal) • Difficulty with verbal and nonverbal communication, social interactions, and leisure or play activities • Limited interests • Repetitive behaviors and a tendency to repeat actions over and over again

continues

TABLE 4.1   DESCRIPTIONS AND CHARACTERISTICS OF SELECT INTELLECTUAL AND DEVELOPMENTAL DISABILITIES (CONT.)

GENERAL DESCRIPTION	COMMON FEATURES OR CHARACTERISTICS
AUTISM SPECTRUM DISORDER (ASD) (CONT.)	
There are three types of ASD: • Autistic disorder • Pervasive developmental disorder (not otherwise specified) • Asperger disorder	• May exhibit aggressive behavior • A tendency to wander or elope; accidental injury because of failure to recognize danger • Sleep problems and irritability. A tendency to repeat or echo words or phrases said to them, or to repeat words or phrases in place of normal language • Difficulty functioning in school, work, and other areas of life • Prefer not to be held or touched • Unable to adjust to new settings, routines, or schedules • Difficulty expressing their needs using typical words or motions • Very sensitive to the environment (lighting, noise, clutter)
CEREBRAL PALSY (CP)	
A group of neurologic disorders that affect a person's ability to move and maintain balance and posture. CP is the most common motor disability in childhood and occurs in 1 in 345 children in the US. It is estimated that there are more than 1 million adults living with CP in the US (Yi, Jung, & Bang, 2019). There are three main kinds of CP: • Spastic CP (increased muscle tone with stiffness and lack of control of muscles)	• Symptoms can range from mild (awkward gait) to moderate (able to walk with special equipment) to severe (unable to walk at all and require lifelong care). • Orthopedic issues may cause poor balance, muscle tone, posture, and reflexes in children. • Everyday tasks may require as much as 3 to 5 times more energy than for people without CP. • Speech is often affected and difficult to understand. • Additional impairments are common and may include cognitive impairment.

- Dyskinetic CP (uncontrollable movement of muscles; affects talking, sucking, and swallowing)

Ataxic CP (impaired balance and coordination) In addition, there are mixed forms of CP, with symptoms of both spastic and dyskinetic CP.

- Mental health disorders are not unusual and warrant screening and treatment.
- Those with cerebral palsy have increased likelihood of pain; fatigue; osteoarthritis; osteoporosis; loss of muscle mass, strength, and endurance; increased spasticity; decreased walking ability; and overuse syndrome with aging
- Those with cerebral palsy may begin to use mobility aids, such as wheelchair or crutches, with aging.

DOWN SYNDROME (DS)

The most common genetic cause of intellectual disability. DS occurs in 1 in 700 children in the US. There are wide estimates of the number of people in the US with Down syndrome, ranging from 250,000 to 400,000 (Presson et al., 2013).

- Physical and cognitive issues
- Characterized by intellectual impairment
- 50% of those with DS are born with a congenital heart defect.
- 75% of those with DS have some hearing loss.
- Ear and eye infections
- Thyroid disorders
- Neck pain, paresthesia, weakness, or signs of compression of the spinal cord due to instability of the craniovertebral junction
- High risk of Alzheimer's dementia with aging

FETAL ALCOHOL SPECTRUM DISORDER (FASD)

A group of conditions that can occur in a person whose mother drank alcohol during pregnancy. FASD occurs in 0.2 to 1.5 of 1,000 infants and 6 to 9 of 1,000 school-age children. FASD is the leading cause of acquired ID and is preventable.

- Preventable if mother does not consume alcohol or stops its consumption during pregnancy
- Can involve physical, behavioral, learning, memory, attention-span, communication, vision, or hearing impairments
- Can be characterized by abnormal facial features, growth problems, and central nervous system (CNS) problems

CDC, n.d.-a, n.d.-c, n.d.-d,, n.d.-e,, n.d.-g

A COMMON EXAMPLE OF IDD: AUTISM SPECTRUM DISORDER

Autism spectrum disorder (ASD) is a neurological developmental disability that generally appears before the age of 3 and lasts throughout life, although symptoms and their severity can change over time (National Institute on Deafness and Other Communication Disorders, 2016). ASD is characterized by significant social, communication, and behavioral issues. The prevalence of ASD is now estimated to be 1 in 59 children (CDC, 2018) and has increased in recent years. It occurs in every racial and ethnic group and across all socioeconomic levels. Its prevalence is significantly higher in boys than girls. Children born to older parents are at greater risk for having ASD, as are those with a sibling with ASD. Although the cause of ASD is unknown, there is some support for genetics and environment being contributing factors.

Three types of ASD have been identified:

- **Autistic disorder:** This bio-neurological developmental disability generally appears before the age of 3 and typically affects social interaction, communication skills, and cognitive function. Individuals with autistic disorder typically have difficulties interacting with others and may exhibit repetitive or stereotyped behaviors (repeating the same words, phrases, or actions in the same order), prefer to play alone, display no interest in the activities of others, and avoid engaging their parents.

- **Pervasive developmental disorder (not otherwise specified):** People with this condition have some but not all of the features that typically characterize autism. The severity of symptoms and behaviors varies widely.

- **Asperger disorder:** People with Asperger disorder often have difficulty with social interactions and prefer following a routine with little variation. However, they often have strong verbal language skills and intellectual abilities.

Some people with ASD are considered "high functioning" and can, with early treatment and intervention, succeed in school and obtain employment. Others have more severe symptoms and require substantial support and assistance to perform even basic functions and activities of living. Some people with ASD have high intelligence levels, while others have low levels. Activities that alter their routine may be met with anger and emotional outbursts. Many people with ASD do not want to be held or even touched. They often react negatively to sensory input, such as bright lights, noise, crowds, and cluttered environments.

One of the most common characteristics of ASD is difficulty communicating and interacting with others. Some people with ASD are nonverbal, although they may be able to communicate in other ways. Some children with ASD have delayed speech and language skills; others exhibit no verbal language skills. Some have fluent speech, but their speech may be awkward, inappropriate, and often repetitive. They may repeat phrases or give answers that are unrelated to questions asked of them. Speech of people with ASD is often flat or robot-like, or it may be sing-song in nature. They may talk about only a narrow range of favorite topics, with little regard for the interests of the person to whom they are speaking. Those with ASD might not respond to others speaking or respond to their own name. This has often led to them being referred for evaluation for hearing problems. Some children with ASD never develop speech and language skills, but they may be able to learn to communicate using gestures, sign language, picture boards, or electronic devices. People with ASD often have a hard time using and interpreting gestures, body language, tone of voice, or facial expressions. They often avoid eye contact with others.

Because of the social, communication, and behavioral issues associated with ASD, healthcare visits may create challenges for both the person with ASD and healthcare professionals, who often have little knowledge or experience interacting with people with this disability. Strategies to make health-related appointments and hospital stays as stress-free as possible include the following:

- Determine how the individual communicates best (e.g., picture boards, electronic devices, verbally).
- Allow the person sufficient time to use that communication method.
- Position yourself so you are visible to the person with ASD.
- Be very specific.
- Avoid using figures of speech.
- Ask concrete questions.
- Avoid asking more than one question at a time.
- Avoid bright lights and noisy environments.
- Avoid unnecessary touching.
- If you must touch the person, let him or her know before doing so.
- Explain the steps and sequence of what will take place, using diagrams, pictures, or models if needed.
- Use distraction if needed to enable the person to participate in activities such as diagnostic testing or drawing blood for testing.

CARING FOR PEOPLE WITH INTELLECTUAL AND DEVELOPMENTAL DISABILITY

Nurses who specialize in caring for individuals with intellectual and developmental disabilities have a high level of expertise in caring for this population (Developmental Disabilities Nurses Association [DDNA], 2020). However, all nurses and other healthcare providers, regardless of healthcare setting, need to have a level of competence and comfort to be able to provide quality care to people with intellectual and developmental disabilities.

People with severe intellectual and developmental disabilities require healthcare that considers their health issues in the context of their disability. However, their care should not focus on the disability to the exclusion of other issues. In other words, the patient's disability should not be the healthcare provider's only focus, but the nature of the disability will influence the care needs of the person. A relationship-based, person-centered, holistic, and lifespan approach to care is essential.

It is important to consider the implications of intellectual and development disabilities on the care that is or should be provided to promote maximum health and well-being.

As discussed in previous chapters, negative attitudes about people with disability on the part of healthcare providers are a potential barrier to quality care. People with IDD are often viewed more negatively by healthcare professionals than those without disability and those with other types of disability. Healthcare professionals often assume that people with IDD are unable to learn, participate in their own care, understand and make informed decisions, or comprehend what is expected or asked of them. Healthcare providers often underestimate the abilities of people with IDD and their interest in maximizing their level of health (Sisirak et al., 2016).

Because IDDs often occur together, nurses and other healthcare professionals will likely interact with people who have developmental disabilities that affect both intellectual and physical function.

An important area of health that is often neglected or dismissed by healthcare professionals in the care of individuals with IDD relates to sexuality, reproductive rights, and access to family-planning care. Individuals with IDD often experience barriers to contraception, preconception counseling, and pregnancy because of disapproval on the part of family members or caregivers and negative attitudes of healthcare providers. Individuals with IDD have the right to make decisions about these issues, which is consistent with their right to self-determination (American Nurses Association, 2019) and the promotion of their quality of life.

Most people facing hospitalization or obtaining care in any healthcare setting are anxious about what may be done to them during their stay and fearful of negative outcomes. People with IDD facing planned hospital stays or clinic or office appointments, as well as those presenting in emergency department settings, are often even more anxious and fearful. For example, they may be anxious about being separated from family members or other trusted support people, be unsure about what to expect, and recall previous adverse or traumatic healthcare or life experiences. Previous negative hospital experiences may contribute to high anxiety and stress levels (Iacono, Bigby, Unsworth, Douglas, & Fitzpatrick, 2014). Although it's not always possible to anticipate the needs of people with IDD prior to healthcare visits or hospital stays, planning in advance to minimize their fears and negative responses can make these experiences more successful and less stressful for all. Preparing materials ahead of time—such as materials for the purposes of distraction and relaxation, as well as booklets with specific information about relevant procedures (presented in simple language and picture formats)—may help enable people with IDDs to cope (Ailey & Hart, 2012).

During initial encounters with people with IDD in any health setting, nurses should conduct a basic head-to-toe assessment to identify immediate or acute issues that may compromise their health and well-being—before obtaining an extensive history. Persons with IDD may have multiple physical needs that must be considered and promptly addressed. For example, the patient may have severe pain or be dehydrated. Or, a patient with a tracheostomy or at risk for aspiration may require immediate attention to ensure the airway is protected. However, even if there are acute issues that must be addressed immediately, nurses and other healthcare providers must not lose sight of the fact that the patient has emotional needs—even if the person is not as responsive as patients without IDDs might be.

In addition to conducting an assessment to identify immediate or acute health issues, healthcare professionals should determine what communication approaches the person is accustomed to using, and to use those approaches. (For more information on communication strategies, see Chapter 3.) Many people with IDD who have impaired communication often become proficient at alternate methods of communication. Thus, it may be appropriate to ask family members or other caregivers what method of communication is effective in interacting with the person with IDD, to use that method yourself, and to inform all other relevant healthcare personnel accordingly. Critically, if patients with IDD are able to communicate using alternative approaches (e.g., picture boards, typed notes, etc.), then adequate time must be provided for them to do so. Reasonable accommodations must be made to ensure quality, person-centered care. People with IDD may bring a health passport (see the "Resources" sidebar at the end of this chapter) with them to their health visit or hospital stay that summarizes information about them; these documents are often helpful to nurses and other healthcare professionals in their assessment and communication with those with IDD.

Although it may be necessary to ask family and other caregivers about a person's preferred methods of communication, all subsequent conversations should be conducted directly with the person with IDD rather than family members or others.

Healthcare providers should assume that individuals—no matter how severe their disability—are able to understand what is being said, even if they are unable to respond. Although providers may ask family members for information, they should not be considered the sole decision-maker. Further, healthcare providers should not rely on family members to provide care to loved ones with IDD who are hospitalized. On the subject of family members, although a person with IDD may be the primary focus, that person's family members also require attention and care. Often, a family member is the sole caretaker and protector of people with IDD. So, family members are often quite concerned about what care their loved ones will receive from healthcare professionals, whether they will be treated with sensitive and appropriate care, and whether their needs will be adequately addressed.

> Persons with disability and their family members are usually the most knowledgeable experts about the person's IDD. Healthcare providers must obtain their input and listen to them.

Persons with severe or profound disability may have multiple physical and emotional needs. People with IDD who have multiple chronic health conditions are twice as likely to have complications when hospitalized and four times as likely to experience complications after surgical procedures. Because of this increased risk of complications—for example, hospital-acquired infections and skin breakdown, falls, and medication errors, including drug interactions—and resulting prolonged lengths of stay (Ailey, Johnson, Fogg, & Friese, 2015), nurses and other healthcare professionals must be diligent in monitoring those with IDD for complications and to be proactive in preventing them.

Additional tips for caring for persons with IDD include the following:

- Minimize noise in the healthcare setting.

- Maintain a peaceful, calm environment to reduce patient stress.

- Allow adequate time and support for them to carry out self-care tasks they are accustomed to doing at home.

- Inform other staff and departments if the person is scheduled for procedures or testing.

- Accompany the person to other units to provide a familiar face.

- Schedule procedures early in the morning to minimize stress and wait times.

- Address the need for preventive healthcare and health promotion, such as regular dental care, health screenings (e.g., mammogram, Pap smear, bone density testing), and physical activity (appropriate for the person).

- Address concerns related to sexuality, reproductive care, and pregnancy. Healthcare providers who have little knowledge or experience working with people with IDD often ignore these issues.

- Because of the high likelihood of poor dental and oral health, do not ignore this aspect of care. Work with the person and family to determine what works best to ensure oral health.

- Provide accessible equipment as needed (e.g., lifts for wheelchair transfers, adjustable exam tables, a wheelchair scale).

- Provide physical assistance to transfer the person from a chair or wheelchair to the exam table and weight scales. Ensure the safety for all during transfers.

Time and patience are needed when caring for patients with intellectual or developmental disability—even in a hectic hospital or clinic setting.

PRACTICE STANDARDS OF DEVELOPMENTAL DISABILITY NURSING

The Practice Standards of Developmental Disabilities Nursing Practice were developed by the Developmental Disabilities Nurses Association (DDNA) for nurses who specialize in caring for people with developmental disability (2020). These standards provide an overview of expectations of nurses and provide a framework and guide to support quality care of people with developmental disabilities in any setting.

Broadly, DDNA identified the following as important expectations of all nurses caring for people with developmental disability:

- Establishing a therapeutic relationship with persons with developmental disability

- Evaluating the person's strengths and challenges in self-direction of care, capacity for independent living, and relationship with others

- Assessing growth and development milestones, use of medications and treatments, bio-psychosocial status, and use of/need for prosthesis and assistive technology

- Assessing the person's daily living patterns (e.g., nutrition and eating, sleep and rest, hygiene and grooming, elimination), functional status (e.g., ability to communicate, toilet, dress, function, mobility), level of understanding to make personal health decisions, and self-medication capabilities

- Assessing behavioral considerations that may affect daily living patterns and functional status

- Encouraging self-advocacy and opportunities to participate in their healthcare decisions, and serving as the person's advocate when necessary

- Implementing a plan of care to promote, maintain, or restore wellness; prevent illness; or provide appropriate end-of-life care

- Assessing and addressing the person's educational needs and those of their family, support team, public at large, and healthcare providers

- Collaborating with the person, family, other supports, and members of the interdisciplinary healthcare team to ensure a person-centered approach toward high-quality care and to promote optimal health and well-being

- Contributing to education and research to improve the evidence base of care for people with developmental disability across the life span

EDUCATING NURSES TO CARE FOR PEOPLE WITH INTELLECTUAL AND DEVELOPMENTAL DISABILITY

As discussed in Chapter 1, there have been numerous calls to address healthcare professionals' lack of knowledge, experience, and expertise in caring for people with disability (including those with IDD). Although nothing will replace actual hands-on interaction and experience of caring for people with IDD, other strategies have been implemented to prepare students in the healthcare professions to provide quality care to this population. Strategies to teach nurses and other healthcare providers about intellectual and developmental disability include the following:

- Add content, modules, or courses on IDD to existing curriculum components in classroom, simulation, home care, and clinical experiences.

- Assign students to read and report on written narratives of people with IDD.

- Establish collaborative relationships with agencies and healthcare facilities that provide care and services to people with IDD (e.g., Special Olympics, The Arc, Association of University Centers on Disability [AUCD]).

- Initiate clinical sites for and with people with IDD and their families for student clinical assignments and visits. (Provide relevant education to students before their first assignment to sites.)

- Identify community agencies with populations of people with IDD to demonstrate for students the ability of people with IDD to participate in activities, work, and school.

- Invite adults with IDD as panelists to talk about their healthcare and health-related experiences in classroom settings with students.

- Explore the inclusion of people with IDD as standardized patients in simulations. Provide training so that expectations are clear to those with IDD, faculty, staff, and students.

Only people with IDD—not actors—should serve as IDD standardized patients. This ensures authentic experiences and prevents stereotyping.

- Build on existing classroom, simulation, home care, and clinical experiences by adding case studies of people with IDD (e.g., add persons with IDD to case studies and simulations currently in use).

- Model positive attitudes toward persons with IDD, behaviors, and skills for students.

- Use available resources to better teach students about IDD (see the following sidebar).

- Assign students to identify modifications to patient teaching plans and strategies to accommodate people with varying types and severity of IDD.

- Assign students to develop teaching materials for family caregivers of persons with IDD and those with IDD with different levels of health literacy and communication methods.

- Explore other campus resources, personnel, and faculty who have expertise/experience with people with disability.

- Explore your own creative and innovative approaches to addressing IDD in curriculum. Focus on the day-to-day lives of those affected rather than limiting your focus to acute care issues in hospital settings.

- Participate in lectures, programs, and courses (if available) on university or college campuses that address diversity or disability issues.

- Identify and collaborate with others on campus with a focus on people with disability (e.g., Disabilities Services, Student Services, or student groups) to identify shared interests and provide mutual support.

- Become active in activities that support individuals with intellectual and developmental disability (i.e., Special Olympics) or disability-related organizations in your city or state or on campus to increase visibility and recognition of the need to ensure that all people, including those with intellectual and developmental disability, receive appropriate education, healthcare, and services.

- Establish a relationship with a person with an intellectual or developmental disability in their own environment as well as in a healthcare setting to learn about their everyday issues, challenges, and accomplishments.

RESOURCES TO TEACH HEALTHCARE PROVIDERS ABOUT INTELLECTUAL AND DEVELOPMENTAL DISABILITY

- **AASPIRE Healthcare Toolkit (https://autismandhealth.org):** This provides resources developed to improve healthcare for adults with autism spectrum disorder.

- **Advancing Care Excellence for Persons with Disabilities (ACE.D):** Communicating with People with Disabilities (http://www.nln.org/professional-development-programs/teaching-resources/ace-d/additional-resources/communicating-with-people-with-disabilities): Part of the Advancing Care Excellence series produced by the National League for Nursing, this resource provides general recommendations for communicating with and providing care for people with a variety of disabilities.

- **Advancing Care Excellence Pediatrics (ACE.P):** Damon McAdam Case Study (http://www.nln.org/professional-development-programs/teaching-resources/ace-p/unfolding-cases/damon-mcadam): Part of the Advancing Care Excellence series produced by the National League for Nursing, this is an unfolding case study of a 2½-year-old child with autism spectrum disorder. The case study and other teaching materials are available on the NLN site and are free to faculty.

- **American Academy for Cerebral Palsy and Developmental Medicine Fact Sheets (https://www.aacpdm.org/publications/fact-sheets):** This website contains multiple fact sheets relevant to the care of persons with CP.

- **American Academy of Developmental Medicine and Dentistry (AADMD) (https://www.aadmd.org):** This website includes resources on IDD, such as educational programs and webinars, including a training program on IDD for primary care nurse practitioners.

- **Autism Speaks: Autism and the Doctor Visit: Communication Tips for Success (https://www.autismspeaks.org/expert-opinion/ autism-and-doctor-visit-communication-tips-success):** This resource provides suggestions for healthcare providers to communicate with people with ASD.

- **Centers for Disease Control and Prevention (CDC): Disability and Health Promotion (https://www.cdc.gov/ncbddd/ disabilityandhealth/index.html):** This resource provides an overview of intellectual and developmental disabilities and details about many specific disabilities (such as Down syndrome).

- **Centers for Disease Control and Prevention (CDC): Facts About Developmental Disabilities (https://www.cdc.gov/ncbddd/ developmentaldisabilities/facts.html):** This resource includes information about developmental milestones, monitoring and screening, causes and risk factors, and more.

- **Centre for Developmental Health Victoria: CDDH Fact Sheet: Working with People with Intellectual Disabilities in Healthcare Settings (https://www.ideas.org.au/uploads/resources/404/working-with-people-with-intellectual-disabilities-in-health-care.pdf):** This fact sheet provides very useful information for healthcare professionals and family caregivers.

- **Developmental Disabilities Nurses Association (https://ddna.org):** This nursing specialty organization provides advocacy, education, and support for nurses who provide services to persons with developmental disabilities, as well as opportunities for certification.

- **The Golisano Institute for Developmental Disability Nursing (GIDDN) at St. John Fisher College (https://www.sjfc.edu/ institutes/golisano-institute/):** This website includes resources and educational materials that address the healthcare of individuals with developmental disabilities.

- **Health Care for Adults with Intellectual and Developmental Disabilities Toolkit for Primary Care Providers: Communicating Effectively (https://iddtoolkit.vkcsites.org/general-issues/ communicating-effectively):** This resource provides suggestions for effective communication with people with intellectual and developmental disability, assessment of individuals with IDD, assessment forms, resources, and tip sheets for a variety of issues.

continues

- **Health Passport (http://flfcic.fmhi.usf.edu/docs/FCIC_Health_ Passport_Form_Typeable_English.pdf):** This health passport is a widely available example of a document that can be completed by/with persons with IDD and brought to the ED/hospital/clinic to help healthcare providers in their assessments and communications with the person. Some hospital systems or community-based IDD agencies may have developed their own health passports.

- **Intellectual and Developmental Disabilities Nursing: Scope and Standards of Practice by the American Nurses Association (the American Nurses Association, 2004):** This book provides information about standards of practice for nurses specializing in intellectual and developmental disabilities.

- **Intellectual Disabilities at Your Fingertips: A Health Care Resource by Dr. Carl V. Tyler and Steve Baker (High Tide Press, 2009):** This pocket-sized resource provides important details about IDD in general and many specific types of IDD. It is useful for clinicians in any healthcare setting.

- **MOIRA: A Quick Reference Guide to Hospital Care for People with a Disability (https://cddh.monashhealth.org/wp-content/ uploads/2017/01/hospital-care.pdf):** This is a useful guide for caring for patients with disability, beginning with an assessment checklist to guide care.

- **National Institute of Dental and Craniofacial Research: Practical Oral Care for People with Developmental Disabilities: Dental Care Every Day: A Caregiver's Guide (https://www.nidcr.nih.gov/sites/default/ files/2018-10/dental-care-everyday.pdf):** This is one of a series of booklets for oral care for people with different types of intellectual and developmental disability for providing and assisting with oral care and preparation for dental visits.

- **National Institute of Neurological Disorders and Stroke: Autism Spectrum Disorder Fact Sheet (https://www.ninds.nih.gov/ Disorders/Patient-Caregiver-Education/Fact-Sheets/Autism-Spectrum-Disorder-Fact-Sheet):** This resource provides a succinct description of autism spectrum disorder and answers many questions about it.

- **National Task Group (NTG) on Intellectual Disabilities and Dementia Practices (https://www.the-ntg.org/):** Affiliated with the American Academy of Developmental Medicine and Dentistry, this task group advocates for people with intellectual disabilities and their families who are affected by Alzheimer's disease and dementias and provides educational workshops and publications.
- **None of Us Want to Stand Still (www.healthmattersprogram.org):** A documentary made in partnership with Rush University and Georgetown University Center for Excellence in Developmental Disability; advocates with IDD discuss their healthcare experiences.
- **Ohio Disability and Health Program/Disability Healthcare Training (https://nisonger.osu.edu/education-training/ohio-disability-health-program/disability-healthcare-training/):** This online training resource is designed to increase healthcare providers' competence in developmental disabilities and addresses healthcare access for people with disabilities. The one-hour session is approved for continuing education by the Centers for Disease Control and Prevention for physicians, nurses, certified health education specialists, and other health professionals.
- **"Primary Care of Adults with Developmental Disabilities" by Sullivan, et al. (https://pubmed.ncbi.nlm.nih.gov/21571716/):** This article discusses Canadian clinical practice guidelines on primary care of adults with IDD. The guidelines are appropriate for any setting and any level of healthcare.
- **Special Olympics: Inclusive Health Principles and Strategies (https://inclusivehealth.specialolympics.org/resources/tools/inclusive-health-principles-and-strategies):** This resource includes information on principles and strategies to ensure the full and sustainable inclusion of people with IDD in health policies and laws, programming, services, education and training programs, research, and funding streams.

SUMMARY

This chapter addressed intellectual and developmental disability. It identified major characteristics of IDD as well as the wide and varied scope of intellectual and developmental disabilities. The chapter addressed the effects of these disabilities on health and healthcare as well as secondary conditions associated with IDD. It also discussed the role of nurses in caring for people with IDD across settings and the need for all healthcare professionals to be prepared to provide sensitive and appropriate, high-quality care for this population. The chapter also covered the importance of communication with individuals with IDD. This included a discussion of matching communication methods to preferences of those with IDD, and the recognition that many individuals with IDD are successful and effective advocates for themselves and others.

Ways to promote the health of and improve the quality of healthcare for individuals with IDD were discussed. Important considerations for all healthcare providers interacting with individuals with IDD were identified, along with multiple resources for caring for people with IDD. Strategies to teach nurses and nursing students about intellectual and developmental disabilities were suggested, along with examples of resources that can be used to ensure that tomorrow's nurses and other healthcare professionals are prepared to provide that care.

REFERENCES

Ailey, S. H., & Hart, R. (2012). Comprehensive program to support patients and staff improves hospital experience for adult patients with intellectual and developmental disabilities at Rush University Medical Center. Washington, D.C.: U.S. Department of Health & Human Services, Agency for Healthcare Research and Quality.

Ailey, S. H., Johnson, T. J., Fogg, L., & Friese, T. R. (2015). Factors related to complications among adult patients with intellectual disabilities hospitalized at an academic medical center. *Intellectual and Developmental Disabilities, 53*(2), 114–119. doi: 10.1352/1934-9556-53.2.114

Ailey, S. H., & Melich-Munyan, T. (2010). Mental and behavioral health disorders in individuals with intellectual and developmental disabilities (pp. 257–276). In C. L. Betz & W. M. Nehring (Eds.). *Nursing care for individuals with intellectual and developmental disabilities: An integrated approach.* Baltimore, MD: Brookes Publishing.

American Nurses Association. (2019). Nurse's role in providing ethically and developmentally appropriate care to people with intellectual and developmental disabilities. Retrieved from https://www.nursingworld.org/~4ab16d/globalassets/practiceandpolicy/ nursing-excellence/ana-position-statements/social-causes-and-health-care/nurses-role-in-providing-ethically-and-developmentally-appropriate-care-to-people-with-intellectual-and-developmental-disabilities.pdf

The ARC. (2014). Self-advocacy. Retrieved from https://thearc.org/wp-content/uploads/2019/08/16-117-The-Arcs-Position-Statements_B9_Self-Advocacy-1.pdf

Auberry, K. (2018). Intellectual and developmental disability nursing: Current challenges in the USA. *Nursing: Research and Reviews, 8,* 23–28.

Betz, C. L., & Nehring, W. M. (2010). Nursing care for individuals with intellectual and developmental disabilities: An integrated approach. Baltimore, MD: Paul H. Brooks, Inc.

Braun, K. V., Christensen, D., Doernberg, N., Schieve, L., Rice, C., Wiggins, L., … & Yeargin-Allsopp, M. (2015). Trends in the prevalence of autism spectrum disorder, cerebral palsy, hearing loss, intellectual disability, and vision impairment, metropolitan Atlanta, 1991–2010. *PLoS ONE, 10*(4), e0124120. doi:10.1371/journal.pone.0124120

Centers for Disease Control and Prevention. (n.d.-a). Attention-deficit/hyperactivity disorder (ADHD). Retrieved from https://www.nimh.nih.gov/health/statistics/attention-deficit-hyperactivity-disorder-adhd.shtml

Centers for Disease Control and Prevention. (n.d.-b). CDC's developmental milestones. Retrieved from https://www.cdc.gov/ncbddd/actearly/milestones/index.html

Centers for Disease Control and Prevention. (n.d.-c). Cerebral palsy (CP). Retrieved from https://www.cdc.gov/ncbddd/cp/index.html

Centers for Disease Control and Prevention. (n.d.-d). Data and statistics on Down syndrome. Retrieved from https://www.cdc.gov/ncbddd/birthdefects/downsyndrome/data.html

Centers for Disease Control and Prevention (n.d.-e). Facts about intellectual disability. Retrieved from https://www.cdc.gov/ncbddd/developmentaldisabilities/facts-about-intellectual-disability.html

Centers for Disease Control and Prevention. (n.d.-e). Fetal alcohol spectrum disorders (FASDs). Retrieved from https://www.cdc.gov/ncbddd/fasd/index.html

Centers for Disease Control and Prevention. (n.d.-g). Key findings: CDC releases first estimates of the number of adults living with autism spectrum disorder in the United States. Retrieved from https://www.cdc.gov/ncbddd/autism/features/adults-living-with-autism-spectrum-disorder.html

Centers for Disease Control and Prevention. (n.d.-h). Key findings: Trends in the prevalence of developmental disabilities in U.S. children, 1997–2008. Retrieved from https://www.cdc.gov/ncbddd/developmentaldisabilities/features/birthdefects-dd-keyfindings.html

Centers for Disease Control and Prevention. (2018). Prevalence of autism spectrum disorder among children aged 8 years—Autism and developmental disabilities monitoring network, 11 sites, United States, 2014. *Morbidity and Mortality Weekly Report, 67*(6), 1–23.

Chiurazzi, P., & Pirozzi, F. (2016). Advances in understanding—Genetic basis of intellectual disability. *F1000 Research, 7*(5), 599. doi:10.12688/f1000research.7134.1

Developmental Disabilities Nurses Association. (2020). Practice standards of developmental disabilities nursing practice. Joliet, IL: High Tide Press.

Fisher, K. (2004). Health disparities and mental retardation. *Journal of Nursing Scholarship. 36*(1), 48–53. https://doi.org/10.1111/j.1547-5069.2004.04010.x

Fisher K. (2012). Is there anything to smile about? A review of oral care for individuals with intellectual and developmental disabilities. *Nursing Research and Practice, 2012,* 860692. https://doi.org/10.1155/2012/860692

Gernsbacher, M. A., Raimond, A. R., Balinghasay, M. T., & Boston, J. S. (2016). "Special needs" is an ineffective euphemism. *Cognitive Research: Principles and Implications 1*(1), 29. doi:10.1186/s41235-016-0025-4

Hahn, J. E., Gray, J., McCallion, P., Ronneberg, C. R., Stancliffe, R. J., Heller, T., ... Janicki, M. P. (2016). Transition in aging: Health, retirement and later life: Review of research, practice, and policy. In *Critical issues in intellectual and developmental disabilities: Contemporary research, practice, and policy* (pp. 149–174). Washington, D.C.: American Association on Intellectual and Developmental Disabilities.

Harris, J. C. (2013). New terminology for mental retardation in DSM-5 and ICD-11. *Current Opinion in Psychiatry, 26*(3), 260–262.

Hughes, K., Bellis, M. A., Jones, L., Wood, S., Bates, G., Eckley, L., ... Officer, A. (2012). Prevalence and risk of violence against adults with disabilities: A systematic review and meta-analysis of observational studies. *The Lancet, 379*(9,826), 1,621–1,629. doi: 10.1016/S0140-6736(11)61851-5

Iacono, T., Bigby, C., Unsworth, C., Douglas, J. & Fitzpatrick, P. (2014). A systematic review of hospital experiences of people with intellectual disability. *BMC Health Services Research,* 2014, 14:505 http://www.biomedcentral.com/1472-6963/14/505

Larson, S. A., Eschenbacher, H., Anderson, L. L. L., Taylor, B., Pettingell, S. L., Hewitt, A. S., ... Bourne, M. L. (2018). In-home and residential supports and services for persons with intellectual or developmental disabilities: Status and trends through 2018. Minneapolis, MN: University of Minnesota Institute on Community Integration.

Lauer, E., & McCallion, P. (2015). Mortality of people with intellectual and developmental disabilities from select US state disability service systems and medical claims data. *Journal of Applied Research in Intellectual Disabilities. 28*(5), 394–405. doi:10.1111/jar.12191

Marks, B., Sisirak, J., Magallanes, R., Krok, K., & Donohue-Chase, D. (2019). Effectiveness of a HealthMessages peer-to-peer program for people with intellectual and developmental disabilities. *Intellectual and Developmental Disabilities, 57*(3), 242–258. doi:10.1352/1934-9556-57.3.242

McKenzie, K., Milton, M., Smith, G., & Ouellette-Kuntz, H. (2016). Systematic review of the prevalence and incidence of intellectual disabilities: Current trends and issues. *Intellectual Disability, 3,* 104–115. doi:10.1007/s40474-016-0085-7

National Institute on Deafness and Other Communication Disorders. (2016). Autism spectrum disorder: Communication problems in children. Retrieved from https://www.nidcd.nih.gov/health/autism-spectrum-disorder-communication-problems-children

National Institute of Dental and Craniofacial Research. (n.d.). Developmental disabilities & oral health. Retrieved from https://www.nidcr.nih.gov/health-info/developmental-disabilities/more-info

Presson, A. P., Partyka, G., Jensen, K. M., Devine, O. J., Rasmussen, S. A., McCabe, L. L., & McCabe, E. R. B. (2013). Current estimate of Down syndrome population prevalence in the United States. *J Pediatr, 163*(4): 1163–1168. doi:10.1016/j.jpeds.2013.06.013

Rimmer, J. H., Yamaki, K., Lowry, B. M., Wang, E., & Vogel, L. C. (2010). Obesity and obesity-related secondary conditions in adolescents with intellectual/developmental disabilities. *Journal of Intellectual Disability Research, 54*(9), 787–794.

Schalock, R. L., Borthwick-Duffy, S. A., Bradley, V. J., Buntinx, W. H. E., Coulter, D. L., Craig, E. M., ... Yeager, M. H. (2012). *User's guide to intellectual disability: Definition, classification, and systems of supports.* Silver Spring, MD: American Association on Intellectual and Developmental Disabilities.

Shea, S. E. (2012). Intellectual disability (mental retardation). *Pediatrics in Review, 33*(3), 110–121. doi:10.1542/pir.33-3-110

Sisirak, J., Marks, B. A.., Heller, T., Ronneberg, C. R., McDonald, K. E., & Ailey, S. (2016). People with IDD: Health and wellness for all. In *Critical issues in intellectual and developmental disabilities: Contemporary research, practice, and policy* (pp. 109–148). Washington, D.C.: American Association on Intellectual and Developmental Disabilities.

Social Security Administration. (2013). Change in terminology: "Mental retardation" to "intellectual disability." *Federal Register, 78*(148). Retrieved from https://www.govinfo.gov/content/pkg/FR-2013-08-01/pdf/2013-18552.pdf

Stanish, H. I., Curtin, C., Must, A., Phillips, S., Maslin, M., & Bandini, L. G. (2019). Does physical activity differ between youth with and without intellectual disabilities *Disability and Health Journal, 12*(3), 503–508. doi:10.1016/j.dhjo.2019.02.006

Sullivan, W. F., Berg, J. M., Bradley, E., Cheetham, T., Denton, R., Heng, J., ... McMillan, S. (2011). Primary care of adults with developmental disabilities: Canadian consensus guidelines. *Canadian Family Physician, 57*(5), 154–168.

Traci, M. A., Seekins, T., Szalda-Petree, A., & Ravesloot, C. (2002). Assessing secondary conditions among adults with developmental disabilities: A preliminary study. *Mental Retardation, 40*(2), 119–131. doi:10.1352/0047-6765(2002)040<0119:ASCAAW>2.0.CO;2

Trollor, J. N., Salomon, C., & Franklin, C. (2016). Prescribing psychotropic drugs to adults with an intellectual disability. *Australian Prescriber, 39(40)*, 126–130.

US Department of Health and Human Services. (2018). *Physical activity guidelines for Americans,* (2nd ed.). Retrieved from https://www.hhs.gov/fitness/be-active/physical-activity-guidelines-for-americans/index.html

Werner, S., & Swawski, M. (2012). Mental health: Knowledge, attitudes and training of professionals on dual diagnosis of intellectual disability and psychiatric disorder. *Journal of Intellectual Disability Research, 56*(3), 291–304.

World Health Organization. (2011). World report on disability. Retrieved from https://www.who.int/publications/i/item/world-report-on-disability

World Health Organization. (2018). Disability and health. Retrieved from https://www.who.int/news-room/fact-sheets/detail/disability-and-health

Yi, Y. G., Jung, S. H., & Bang, M. S. (2019). Emerging issues in cerebral palsy associated with aging: A physiatrist perspective. *Annals of Rehabilitation Medicine, 43*(3), 241–249. doi:10.5535/arm.2019.43.3.241

Zablotsky, B., Black, L. I., Maenner, M. J., Schieve, L. A., Danielson, M. L., Bitsko, R. H., ... Boyle, C. A. (2019). Prevalence and trends of developmental disabilities among children in the United States: 2009–2017. *Pediatrics, 144*(4), e20190811. doi:10.1542/peds.2019-0811

5
PHYSICAL DISABILITY

INTRODUCTION

Physical disability is often the most visible type of disability. It is difficult *not* to see when someone uses a wheelchair or a mobility aid such as a cane, walker, or crutches, or to notice that someone is missing one or more extremities.

Just as different federal and state agencies define the general term *disability* in different ways, the term *physical disability* has different definitions. One definition, developed by the Independence Care System (2016) based on the Americans with Disabilities Act of 1990, and published in *A Blueprint for Improving Access to Primary Care for Adults with Physical Disabilities*, describes physical disability as a functional limitation (specifically, in mobility) that affects one or more activities of daily living—for example, bathing, toileting, cooking, walking, transferring, or dressing.

Another way of defining or describing disability is by function or functional type based on self-reported difficulties (Centers for Disease Prevention and Control [n.d.-a]. Using this approach, physical disability can be equated to some degree with the following categories (with the first category most closely aligned):

- **Mobility limitations:** Serious difficulty walking or climbing stairs

- **Independent living limitations:** Difficulty doing errands such as shopping or visiting a physician's office alone

- **Self-care limitations:** Difficulty dressing or bathing

In its Survey of Income and Program Participation (SIPP), the US Census Bureau (2014) defined physical disability as follows:

- Requiring the use of a wheelchair, a cane, crutches, or a walker

- Difficulty performing one or more of the following functional activities: seeing, hearing, speaking, lifting/carrying, using stairs, walking, or grasping small objects

- Difficulty with one or more activities of daily living (getting around inside the home, getting in or out of bed or a chair, bathing, dressing, eating, and toileting)

- Difficulty with one or more instrumental activities of daily living (going outside the home, keeping track of money and bills, preparing meals, doing light housework, taking prescription medicines in the right amount at the right time, and using the telephone)

> The functional limitations addressed in the SIPP cover difficulties with hearing, seeing, cognitive activities, ambulatory activities, self-care activities, and independent living activities.

Finally, the terminology used by the Centers for Disease Control and Prevention (CDC) in the National Health Interview Survey (NHIS) demonstrates the complexity of definitions of disability in general and physical disability specifically (CDC, n.d.-b):

- Has limitation of activity (e.g., personal care needs, routine needs, inability to work, limited work, walking, remembering; other physical, mental, or emotional limitations)

- Requires use of special equipment (e.g., cane, wheelchair, special bed, special telephone)

MORE ON THE NHIS

The NHIS, which combines the efforts of multiple agencies and organizations interested in monitoring the health of the nation, includes questions related to the following topics:

- Work limitations
- The need for assistance with tasks related to personal care, such as eating, bathing, dressing, and getting around inside the home
- The need for assistance with routine tasks, such as everyday household chores, shopping or running errands, and doing necessary business

Many of these limitations can occur with physical disability. They may also occur with IDD, IDD combined with physical disability, sensory disability, psychiatric/mental health disability, or aging.

PREVALENCE OF PHYSICAL DISABILITY

Because disability in general and physical disability in particular are defined differently across sources and federal agencies, the estimates of the prevalence of disability and physical disability also differ from one report to another. However, there is general agreement that about one in every four (25.7%) adults in the US has some type of disability. This represents more than 61.4 million people. The percentage of adults with mobility limitations (serious difficulty walking or climbing stairs) has been estimated to be 13.7%. The percentages of the population with independent-living limitations (difficulty doing errands alone) and self-care limitations (difficulty dressing or bathing)—both of which could be due in part to mobility limitations—are estimated to be 6.5% and 3.6%, respectively (Okoro, Hollis, Cyrus, & Griffin-Blake, 2018).

The prevalence of physical disability differs by age group, gender, race, and socioeconomic status. Mobility limitation is most prevalent among middle-aged (18.1%) and older adults (26.9%). Among all age groups, the prevalence of any disability and of each type are higher among women than men, with the exceptions of hearing and self-care limitations (Okoro et al., 2018). The highest prevalence of any disability and of each type of disability occurs among older adults from American Indian/Alaska Native (54.9%), Hispanic (50.5%), and other race/multiracial groups (49.9%). The prevalence of disability increases with poverty level, with lower levels of education, and in the South compared to other regions of the US (Okoro et al., 2018).

People with disability are more likely to be unemployed or underemployed and generally earn less even when they are employed. Both employment and income outcomes worsen with the severity of disability.

CAUSES OF PHYSICAL DISABILITY

Just as definitions of physical disability differ by source, there is also disagreement on the common causes of disability. To some extent, this is due to differences in definitions of disability. But generally, it is safe to say that multiple causes of physical disability exist, and major categories of causes can be identified:

- Acute illness

- Chronic illness

- Trauma

Disabilities can be developmental or acquired. Developmental disabilities that affect physical rather than intellectual function (discussed in Chapter 4) manifest during the developmental years up to the age of 22. Because many children with developmental disabilities that largely affect physical function—such as spina bifida, cerebral palsy, osteogenesis imperfecta, and others—now live full lives well into adulthood and even old age, they also fit most criteria for having a physical disability.

Acquired physical disabilities are those that occur after the developmental years as a result of trauma or acute or chronic illness. Examples of trauma-related acquired physical disabilities include traumatic brain injury, spinal cord injuries, and traumatic loss of extremities (CDC, n.d.-b, n.d.-f). Acquired physical disabilities due to acute or chronic illness include the following (Global Burden of Disease 2017 Disease and Injury Incidence and Prevalence Collaborators, 2018; National Institute of Neurological Disorders and Stroke, 2019; Shulman, 2010; United States Bone and Joint Initiative, 2016; World Health Organization [WHO], 2019):

- Stroke

- Multiple sclerosis (MS)

- Motor neurone diseases such as amyotrophic lateral sclerosis (ALS), progressive muscular atrophy, and post-polio syndrome

- Severe cardiovascular or respiratory diseases that limit one's mobility

- Morbid obesity

- Autoimmune disorders

- Musculoskeletal disorders such as osteoarthritis, rheumatoid arthritis, and skeletal changes or fractures due to osteoporosis

- Diabetes

- Parkinson's disease

This is only a partial list of acquired physical disabilities.

- Cancer

- Amputation of extremities due to chronic health conditions such as diabetes or cancer, or septic shock

CONSEQUENCES OF PHYSICAL DISABILITY

Despite the high visibility of a number of physical disabilities, many individuals with these disabilities report that healthcare settings are often inaccessible, their disability is not considered when they are seeking or receiving healthcare, and healthcare providers often fail to make accommodations to ensure that they receive high-quality healthcare.

Many people with physical disability report that:

- Healthcare settings are often inaccessible.

- Healthcare is difficult to obtain.

- Healthcare providers ignore their disability or do not know how to address the effects of it when members of this population seek or receive healthcare.

- Healthcare providers do not consider the effects of disability with respect to obtaining preventive health screenings or engaging in health promotion activities.

- Healthcare providers often do not make accommodations to ensure that members of this population receive high-quality healthcare.

As a result, people with one or more types of disability are at higher risk of mortality than those without, with those with physical disability having the strongest risk of all (Forman-Hoffman et al., 2015).

Although many types of physical disabilities are obvious, other types are not readily observed by others despite being severely limiting.

The World Health Organization (WHO) (2011, 2015) has identified many physical barriers to healthcare for people with disability. A number of these are specific to people with physical disability. These include the following:

- Inaccessible parking areas at healthcare facilities

- The absence of ramps and curb cuts, or ramps that are too steep

- Steps outside buildings that offer healthcare services that hamper entry

- Steps inside buildings that offer healthcare services that prevent movement from floor to floor

- Narrow doorways that do not accommodate wheelchairs or other mobility devices

- Heavy doors or a lack of automatic doors

- Doorknobs that cannot be used by people with limited hand function

- Inadequate space

- The absence of height-adjustable examination tables, weight scales, and imaging equipment

- A lack of grab bars

- A lack of accessible restrooms

- Reception desks that are too high to permit people in wheelchairs to speak easily with receptionists

- Poor signage

Because of these physical barriers to healthcare facilities, people with mobility difficulties are often unable to obtain healthcare or undergo recommended preventive healthcare screening. For example, cervical cancer screening is difficult if examination tables and diagnostic equipment are not adjustable. Similarly, mammograms are impossible to obtain if equipment does not accommodate women who are unable to stand and maintain difficult positions, or if mammography personnel are not familiar with the accommodations needed for women with physical disability.

As discussed in Chapter 3, negative attitudes and lack of knowledge about disability on the part of healthcare professionals—including nurses—have resulted in myths, misconceptions, and low expectations of people with disability (CDC, n.d.-a). However, a 2012 review of studies found that healthcare students and professionals had generally favorable attitudes toward people with physical disability. This review also revealed that students' attitudes were more favorable than those of professionals in practice, as were attitudes of people who had previous contact with those with physical disability compared to people with little or no previous contact. Casual or social contact with a person with disability was also found to be associated with more favorable attitudes (Satchidanand et al., 2012).

However, even when healthcare professionals' attitudes are generally positive, if they have inadequate knowledge about disability and all that it entails, care for people with physical disability will remain inadequate. To illustrate this point, consider that physical and attitudinal barriers have resulted in the following:

- Many women who use wheelchairs who seek reproductive healthcare report that they are examined in their wheelchairs and have not been weighed for years—even during pregnancy (Long-Bellil, Mitra, Iezzoni, Smeltzer, & Smith, 2017).

- Women with physical and other types of disability indicate that their healthcare providers assume they are asexual (or perhaps believe they should be) (Independence Care System, 2016).

- Obstetrical care providers have turned away women with physical and other types of disability who are interested in becoming pregnant, discouraged them from considering pregnancy, counseled them to terminate their pregnancies, and otherwise ignored their preferences and healthcare needs (Smeltzer, Mitra, Iezzoni, Long-Bellil, & Smith (2016).

- Women with physical and other types of disability have reported receiving little or no information about pregnancy in the context of their disability from healthcare professionals; a dearth of information in childbirth education classes about what they can expect as well as the effects of their disability on labor, delivery, and the postpartum period; no accommodations during the postpartum period; and no assistance planning childcare (Mitra, Long-Bellil, Iezzoni, Smeltzer, & Smith, 2016; Smeltzer, Wint, Ecker, & Iezzoni, 2017).

> Self-determination is a right of all people, including those with disability. Individuals with disability—physical and otherwise—have the right to make decisions about their own lives, including their plans for childbearing. These decisions should not be made for them based on the personal biases of healthcare providers. They also have a right to receive the information they need to make informed decisions about their own care.

Some common health conditions that can be problems for all groups may be more significant for those with physical disability. For example, if people who are wheelchair users become overweight or obese, their ability to use or fit into their wheelchair, to transfer in and out of the chair, and to move about may be hampered.

Health promotion and disease prevention should be part of the healthcare provided to all people to enable them to stay well, active, and part of their family and community. Yet, healthcare professionals often neglect to address these issues with people with disability. For people with disability, health promotion also means treating health problems related to the disability. These problems (also called secondary conditions) can include pain, depression, and a greater risk for other illnesses.

Compounding these problems is a lack of accessible transportation for people with disability in general. (See Chapter 3.) These barriers seem to be particularly burdensome for those with physical disability and may prevent them from accessing healthcare. Although a 2015 report from the National Council on Disability (NCD) indicates that transportation has improved for people with disability since 2005, it also includes nearly 400 recommendations to make every mode of transportation more accessible (NCD, 2015).

Lack of accessible transportation—and more specifically accessible exercise facilities—also affects the health of people with physical disability. This is because it may prevent them from participating in exercise programs. This could in turn contribute to their becoming overweight or obese—limiting their ability to participate in such programs or activities even further.

Despite all this, having a disability does not mean being unhealthy. Although more people with disability do report poor health than those without disability, most people with disability report their health to be good, very good, or excellent. People with disability, including those with severe physical disability, can be healthy and live active, meaningful, and productive lives. Receiving high-quality healthcare contributes to good health and can help prevent or minimize the effects of secondary health conditions or common

There have been efforts to address barriers that impede the ability of people with physical disability to obtain quality healthcare and live their lives to their fullest. However, many barriers remain, despite legal mandates to remove them.

health conditions that affect the rest of the population. Healthcare professionals should encourage all people—with or without disability—to make healthy choices and develop strategies to prevent illness (CDC, n.d.-c).

CONSEQUENCES OF LACK OF ACCESSIBLE HEALTHCARE OF PEOPLE WITH PHYSICAL DISABILITY

Limited access to healthcare for people with physical disability results in a number of consequences. Compared to people without physical disability, people with physical disability have:

- Higher rates of untreated obesity, arthritis, asthma, cardiovascular disease, diabetes, high blood pressure, high cholesterol, and stroke (Forman-Hoffman et al., 2015; Reichard, Stolzle, & Fox, 2011)
- Lower likelihood of receiving preventive health services such as cancer screenings—for example, gynecological exams, mammograms, and colonoscopies (McCarthy et al., 2006; WHO, 2018)
- Lower level of participation in health promotion and disease prevention due to the failure of healthcare providers to attend to these measures in their care for this population (WHO, 2018)
- Lower likelihood of receiving education about birth control measures, risks of unprotected sex and sexually transmitted diseases, and unwanted pregnancy (Sinclair, Taft, Sloan, Stevens, & Krahn, 2015; WHO, 2018)
- Higher risk of pressure ulcers, urinary tract infections, pain, and untreated osteoporosis with increased risk of fractures with falls (WHO, 2015, 2018)
- Lower likelihood of assessment of psychological status; inadequate treatment of depression, anxiety, and stress; and higher risk of physical, verbal, and sexual abuse, personal violence, and other crimes (Forman-Hoffman et al., 2015)
- Higher risk of mortality from cancer because of delayed diagnoses and receipt of less aggressive treatment (Forman-Hoffman et al., 2015; McCarthy et al., 2006; WHO, 2011, 2018)
- Higher risk of hospitalization, morbidity, and mortality due to all causes (Forman-Hoffman et al., 2015; WHO, 2011)

CHARACTERISTICS OF SELECT PHYSICAL DISABILITIES

Physical disabilities can be very diverse. They can result from a wide variety of disabling conditions, ranging from those that begin early in life to those that largely affect older adults. Some physical disabilities change or progress over time. Others remain unchanged from their initial occurrence.

Some physical disabilities are minor in severity—more of an inconvenience than something that has major effects on one's function, life activities, plans, and quality of life. Others are more severe, requiring accommodations to enable affected people to move about, attend school or work, and participate in desired activities with friends, family, and the community. Some physical disabilities may even necessitate round-the-clock care and major technical assistance for survival.

> Many people with physical disability require accommodations that, if implemented, enable them to live full, productive, and meaningful lives.

Table 5.1 lists several physical disabilities and information about each one. Although it includes only a limited number of disabilities, the types of disabling conditions and their characteristics demonstrate the scope of disorders that cause physical disability. The specific characteristics of each condition and how it affects people influence the specific issues related to providing care.

CARING FOR PEOPLE WITH PHYSICAL DISABILITY

Caring for people with physical disability depends on several factors:

- The type of disability and its cause

- The severity of the disability and its impact on health status and other functions and resulting limitations

- The length of time since the onset of the disability and its likely outcome

- The person's psychological and emotional responses to the disability

- The setting in which care is to be provided (primary care, hospital, outpatient, home or community-based)

- The reason the person is seeking care (the primary or immediate health issue may pertain to the disability, or it could be another health issue generally unrelated to the disability)

- The person's ability to cope with and manage the changes in lifestyle and daily life that may occur with disability

- The availability of support from family members or others

- The availability and accessibility of other services

Healthcare professionals should make no assumptions about people with disability and their healthcare needs, their interest in and ability to obtain care and to follow health-related recommendations, and their preferences related to care.

Healthcare providers are often reluctant to ask patients with disability about their disability for fear of distressing them. This is especially true for inexperienced healthcare professionals, including nursing students. As for experienced health professionals, they may fail to discuss a patient's disability because they believe they know all they need to know about it. Or, if the disability is long-standing rather than acute or recent, they might think it is unlikely to be a significant issue in the patient's life or care. However, none of these scenarios is likely to be true. Most people with disability are very well aware that they have a disability and are reassured by healthcare providers acknowledging it. Such providers are more likely to consider how the disability affects the patient's health status and access to healthcare than providers who ignore the disability, fail to notice the disability, or do not consider it in the plan of care.

TABLE 5.1 DESCRIPTIONS AND CHARACTERISTICS OF SELECT PHYSICAL DISABILITIES

GENERAL DESCRIPTION	COMMON FEATURES OR CHARACTERISTICS
MULTIPLE SCLEROSIS (MS)	
An unpredictable, usually progressive disease in which the immune system attacks the myelin covering nerve fibers in central nervous system structures, usually in the brain stem, cerebellum, spinal cord, and optic nerves, as well as the white matter of the brain (Ghasemi, Razavi, & Nikzad, 2017). The severity of MS and resulting disability depend on the magnitude of the immune reaction as well as the location and extent of MS lesions or plaques in the brain. Onset of MS is typically between 20 to 40 years of age, but it can occur in children and older people. MS is the most common disabling neurological disease among young adults and is more common in women. MS affects about 400,000 Americans and 2.5 million people globally. Symptoms can range from relatively mild to profound. Patients with profound symptoms may be unable to walk, write, speak, or swallow. Partial or complete paralysis can occur with severe disease. In some forms of MS (relapsing-remitting MS), symptoms may come and go. In other forms, the course is progressive from the onset of symptoms (primary or secondary progressive types). Exacerbations (attacks) can be mild or severe, depending on the site of MS lesions. Even if attacks are severe, however, recovery to baseline is often possible with adequate treatment and supportive care. Disease-modifying medications are available, but currently most of them target relapsing-remitting forms of MS. Life expectancy is usually normal.	• Optic neuritis with blurred or double vision; can result in blindness. • Fatigue, bladder and bowel dysfunction, paresthesia (tingling and burning sensations), pain, balance problems and lack of coordination, dizziness, muscle weakness or spasms, impaired speech, impaired swallowing • Cognitive dysfunction, impaired executive functioning, decreased ability to concentrate, memory deficits, poor judgment • Depression • Inappropriate laughing or crying (called *pseudobulbar* symptoms)

DIABETES-RELATED DISABILITY

Well-controlled type 2 diabetes itself is not universally considered a disability. However, diabetes that results in complications (e.g., diabetic neuropathy, retinopathy, nephropathy, cardiac disease, and stroke due to microvascular and macrovascular changes) may lead to disability due to vision loss, renal failure, stroke and cardiac dysfunction, and loss of extremities due to amputation. Risk of stroke and heart attack is 2 to 3 times higher in adults with diabetes (American Diabetes Association, 2020a; 2020b; 2020c; Dokken, 2008).

More than 422 million adults have diabetes globally, representing 1 in every 11 people. Diabetes was the seventh leading cause of death globally in 2016 (CDC, n.d.-d).

Complications of diabetes that result in disability are typically present for many years before symptoms occur as vascular changes damage blood vessels and organs.

Although eligible for disability services, those affected may not consider themselves to have a disability.

- Increased likelihood of foot ulcers, infection, and amputation due to neuropathy and decreased vascular supply to the feet and legs
- Vision loss from diabetic retinopathy, a very common cause of blindness in the US
- Increased kidney failure due to diabetic nephropathy
- May be prevented or minimized by control of diabetes and blood glucose levels

SPINAL CORD INJURY

The result of damage to the spinal cord due to external trauma. The most common examples of trauma are vehicle crashes followed by falls. Acts of violence (often gunshot wounds) and sports or recreation activities are also fairly common causes. SCI is the most common cause of paralysis in the US.

More than 17,700 new cases of SCI occur each year. (This number represents those who survived the initial injury.) An estimated 247,000 to 358,000 people in the US live with a SCI. The average age of injury is 43 years, and 78% of new SCIs occur in males (National Spinal Cord Injury Statistical Center, 2018).

- Varies widely in severity and level of injury
- Ability to move and use upper and lower extremities depends on level and severity of injury
- Possible loss of bowel, bladder, and sexual function
- Decreased ability to breathe and to generate cough when injury occurs in the cervical spine or high thoracic level, increasing risk of respiratory problems
- Increased risk of pressure ulcers and joint damage due to lack of sensation

continues

TABLE 5.1 DESCRIPTIONS AND CHARACTERISTICS OF SELECT PHYSICAL DISABILITIES (CONT.)

GENERAL DESCRIPTION	COMMON FEATURES OR CHARACTERISTICS
A complete SCI, in which the spinal cord is severed, results in a total lack of sensory and motor function below the injury. Some motor and sensory function may be retained below the injury with incomplete SCIs.	• Increased risk of autonomic dysreflexia (a potentially life-threatening medical emergency that may occur with SCI at or above T6 level of injury; may be some risk with those with T7 to T10 level of SCI); risk increases with pain, full bladder, urinary tract infection, distended bowel, pressure ulcers, or labor and delivery

AMPUTATION

Absence or loss of body part due to trauma, chronic vascular insufficiency secondary to diabetes or other disorders, infection, bone or muscle loss, septic shock, or congenital factors.	• Affects body image and quality of life
	• Often affects mobility and balance (with lower extremity loss)
More than 2 million people in the US live with limb loss, with 185,000 new amputations each year. (Ziegler-Graham, MacKenzie, Ephraim, Travison, & Brookmeyer, 2008).	• May affect ability to carry out personal activities of daily living (eating, dressing, lifting, grasping, and toileting)
Limitations are determined by the extent of loss (partial versus whole extremity) and the ability of the individual to use assistive devices and prostheses for mobility and other functions.	
Amputation is often life-altering. Even if amputation occurred years ago, the resulting changes in function, and people's responses to those changes, must be considered at every healthcare encounter. It cannot be assumed that individuals have accepted or adjusted to the changes in their body, functions, and life goals because the amputation occurred many years ago.	

DISABILITY DUE TO AMPUTATION OR CONGENITAL ABSENCE OF EXTREMITIES: EXAMPLES FOR ILLUSTRATIVE PURPOSES

It has been estimated that 1 in 190 people in the US is currently living with the loss of one or more extremities. Loss or absence of extremities may be due to diverse causes and occur in diverse circumstances. The circumstances in which loss or absence occurred will have major effects on how people respond to the loss itself; their views, perceptions, and emotional reactions to the resulting disability that occurs; their motivation to participate in rehabilitation; and the extent and speed of their return to previous activities. Examples of various scenarios follow:

- A 29-year-old soldier who recently experienced traumatic amputation of both legs during military deployment has a high likelihood of also having post-traumatic stress disorder (PTSD) and may consider his life completely derailed and his quality of life unacceptable.

- A 55-year-old man who has worked in construction for 30 years who has undergone surgical above-the-knee amputation of one leg because of long-standing, poorly controlled diabetes may experience anger and depression. He may also fear the loss of his other leg and that he will never be able to work again.

- A 32-year-old woman who experienced surgical above-the-elbow amputation of her dominant arm because of bone cancer (osteosarcoma) at the age of 19 who is considering pregnancy after 5 years of marriage may be concerned and anxious about her ability to care for a newborn with her one arm.

- A 64-year-old man who has experienced a below-the-knee amputation because of severe, intractable pain resulting from peripheral arterial disease may express relief after the postoperative pain has resolved and may be eager to get on with his life.

- A 48-year-old woman who was born with a hemipelvectomy who is hospitalized overnight for a hysterectomy may be eager to get up and around after surgery and back to her busy schedule as a parent of three adolescents and as a high-school science teacher.

Because of the diverse circumstances, length of time since the loss occurred, and varied psychological and emotional responses to the loss and the resulting disability, healthcare providers must assess people's responses, current health status beyond the loss of an extremity, and effects of the loss and the resulting disability on other health-related issues such as PTSD, diabetes, pain relief, or plans for pregnancy.

Even if limb loss results in relief of severe, unrelenting pain, most people who experience it require time and support to become accustomed to the change in mobility status and to the loss of independence that will likely follow. In the case of lower extremity loss, they will have to learn new methods of moving from place to place, which may involve use of a wheelchair or assistive mobility aids such as crutches or prostheses. They may also need to learn to use a prosthesis, if they elect to use one, to carry out usual activities such as eating, bathing, dressing, taking care of themselves and others, and working in new ways. In addition, they will need to adjust to the added weight of the prosthesis and the fatigue that often accompanies its initial use. Finally, they may have to rely on others for assistance, support, and understanding as they figure out ways to do the everyday tasks that were once easy and second nature to them.

Healthcare providers must anticipate that people with limb loss may be adjusting to the loss and to changes in physical function that may result. Even if the amputation occurred years ago, the resulting disability must be considered in providing quality, comprehensive care to the individual.

Disability may affect healthcare issues and access to healthcare even if it has been present for decades. For example, forms of cerebral palsy that have been present since birth or early childhood that significantly impair mobility will affect that person's ability to participate in some activities in the absence of accommodations, to obtain preventive health screening, and to participate in health promotion and physical exercise and activities even decades later. Another example might be that of a patient whose leg was amputated many years ago who is diagnosed with congestive heart failure. This new health issue would likely require the patient to weigh himself daily to monitor himself for fluid retention; this patient might require assistance to determine how best to perform this task safely.

It is also important to keep in mind that a patient with a physical disability may experience increasing mobility limitations

The existence of a disability cannot be ignored even if has been present for years.

or other physical issues with aging. For example, a person who has used mobility aids (e.g., crutches or a wheelchair) for decades may experience the consequences of years of repetitive stress on the joints involved in the use of these devices. Overuse injuries in the upper extremities may occur in those who are long-term wheelchair users, particularly those who have used their upper extremities for propelling their wheelchair and transferring to and from their wheelchair.

A disability may necessitate modifications in how healthcare providers conduct histories and physical assessments. For example, the history should address the effect of the disability—even if present for many years—on the patient's day-to-day activities. It should also address the effects of the disability on other health issues as well as the effect of those health issues on the disability. As for the assessment, healthcare providers may need to modify the sequence of steps or use alternate approaches for patients who require assistance to stand, walk, or change positions. Assistance from healthcare staff is essential in these circumstances—for example, in changing positions or in transferring to and from an exam table.

The safety of both the person with disability and assistive personnel is important. Adjustable exam tables and accessible weight scales are essential to ensure quality care for people with disability. Advocating for this equipment may be necessary to ensure its availability.

> When communicating with someone sitting in a chair or wheelchair, it is important for the healthcare provider to sit at the individual's eye level.

Although it is important to consider the effects of disability on people's health status, needs, and care, it is equally important to avoid *overshadowing*—that is, attributing *all* their health issues to the presence of a disability. That being said, it is also essential to be aware that people with physical disability are at risk for secondary conditions related to their disability, as well as for unrelated, general health issues.

People with disability could have other disabling conditions that may or may not be related to their physical disability. These include mental, emotional, and psychological issues such as depression, anxiety, and dementia. Do not assume that a person's physical disability is the only cause of any mental, emotional, or psychological conditions, however—although it might be. Healthcare providers should evaluate and treat these conditions in people with disability the same way they would people without physical disability.

> Omitting aspects of the physical assessment merely because of the presence of physical disability is unacceptable healthcare and may result in lack of detection of health problems that require attention.

> Healthcare providers should address mental, emotional, and psychological conditions that arise in response to disability with appropriate counseling or referrals for psychological services.

To reduce the risk of morbidity and mortality, healthcare professionals should address the acute healthcare needs of people with physical disability as well as their long-term health issues. Lack of preventive health screening may be a factor in higher mortality; thus, access to screening along with appropriate accommodations to ensure accurate results and follow-up care could reduce the premature mortality rate of those with physical disability (Forman-Hoffman et al., 2015).

Many—but not all—of the health issues experienced by people with physical disability are related to complications from immobility or decreased mobility. Even patients who are immobilized for just 24 hours are at increased risk for complications due to immobility, including pressure ulcers, deep vein thrombosis, pneumonia, and urinary tract infections (Wu et al., 2018). People with physical disability that reduces their mobility may be immobilized for even longer periods; thus, healthcare providers must consider the risk for these same complications for this population.

Other health conditions that people with physical disability might experience include contractures and spasm. These may result in pain or injury and should be evaluated and treated accordingly.

People with physical disability often find hospital stays to be frightening. When asked about their experiences during hospital stays, people with physical disability described the following (Smeltzer, Avery, & Haynor, 2012):

- Ineffective communication with members of the nursing staff

- Compromised care

- Negative attitudes on the part of nursing staff

- Fear of leaving the hospital in poorer condition than when they entered

When people with physical disability are hospitalized, it is important for nurses and other healthcare staff and providers to do the following:

- Communicate effectively with them.

- Ask them what their goals and preferences are.

- Consider them the experts on their disability.

- Ask them how best to assist them to move about.

- Provide adequate assistance in moving or transferring to ensure the safety of those with disability and of staff.

- Ensure that any needed assistive devices are readily available and convenient.

Prevention of complications due to immobility is also essential. Although people with disability may be confined to bed only temporarily because of treatments, recent surgery, or acute illness, they are particularly susceptible to complications related to immobility and have a narrow margin of health or safety. So, strategies to minimize complications are essential.

CHARACTERISTICS OF DISABILITY-COMPETENT CARE

A Blueprint for Improving Access to Primary Care for Adults with Physical Disabilities, developed by the Independence Care System (2016), identifies characteristics of disability-competent primary care. These characteristics apply to all healthcare professionals providing care for people with physical disability in any setting:

- Treat every patient as a whole person and an individual, not a diagnosis or condition.

- Identify barriers people with physical disability face in the community and in the healthcare system.

- Focus on optimizing people's health and wellness while supporting their maximum function, independence, and ability to live in the community as they choose.

- Respond to people's physical and clinical needs while also considering their emotional, social, intellectual, and spiritual needs.

- Encourage an interdisciplinary approach, with healthcare professionals collaborating across disciplines and care settings.

EDUCATING NURSES TO CARE FOR PEOPLE WITH PHYSICAL DISABILITY

Following are several strategies to teach nurses, nursing students, and other healthcare professionals about physical disability:

- Add content, modules, or courses on physical disability to existing curriculum components in classroom, simulation, home care, and clinical experiences.

- Assign students to view and write a report on one of the stories about people with disability produced by the Disability Rights Education & Defense Fund (DREDF). These stories can be found here: https://dredf.org/healthcare-stories/index/.

- Establish collaborative relationships with agencies and healthcare facilities that provide care and services to people with physical disability (e.g., adult day care settings and local community-based programs and services).

- Initiate clinical sites for and with people with physical disability and their families for student clinical assignments and visits. (Provide relevant education to students before first assignment to sites.)

- Identify community agencies with populations of people with physical disability to demonstrate for students the ability of people with physical disability to participate in activities, work, and school.

- Invite people with physical disability to participate in lectures and panel discussions to enable students to become comfortable asking about physical disability and to learn firsthand about the health-related experiences of people with physical disability.

- Explore the inclusion of people with physical disability as standardized patients in simulations. Provide training so that expectations are clear to those with physical disability, faculty, staff, and students.

- Build on existing classroom, simulation, home care, and clinical experiences by adding case studies of people with physical disability.

- Model positive attitudes toward persons with physical disability, and appropriate behaviors and skills for students.

- Use available resources to better teach students about physical disability (see the following sidebar).

Only people with physical disability—not actors— should serve as physical disability standardized patients. This ensures authentic experiences and prevents stereo- typing (Smeltzer, Mariani, Ross, de Mange, Meakim, Bruderle, & Nthenge, 2015; Smeltzer et al., 2018).

- Assign students to identify modifications to patient teaching plans and strategies to accommodate people with varying types and severity of physical disabilities.

- Explore other campus resources, personnel, and faculty who have expertise/experience with people with physical disability.

- Assign students to assess their clinical sites and other relevant sites for accessibility using the sample accessibility survey form found in the NYS Health Foundation's *A Blueprint for Improving Access to Primary Care for Adults with Physical Disabilities,* located here: https://nyshealthfoundation.org/wp-content/uploads/2017/12/A_Blueprint_for_Improving_Access_to_Primary_Care_for_Adults_with_Physical_Disabilities.pdf

- Participate in disability studies lectures, programs, and courses (if available) on the university or college campus.

- Identify and collaborate with others on campus with a focus on people with disability (e.g., Disabilities Services or Student Services) to identify shared interests and provide mutual support.

- Become active in disability-related organizations in your city or state or on campus to increase visibility and recognition of the need to ensure that all people, including those with physical disability, receive appropriate education, healthcare, and services.

- Establish a relationship with people with physical disability in their own environment as well as in a healthcare setting to learn about their everyday issues, challenges, and accomplishments.

- Explore your own creative and innovative approaches to addressing physical disability in curriculum. Focus on the day-to-day lives of those affected rather than limiting your focus to acute care issues in hospital settings.

RESOURCES TO TEACH HEALTHCARE PROVIDERS ABOUT PHYSICAL DISABILITY

- **Advancing Care Excellence for Persons with Disabilities (ACE.D): Communicating with People with Disabilities (http://www.nln.org/professional-development-programs/teaching-resources/ace-d/additional-resources/communicating-with-people-with-disabilities):** Part of the Advancing Care Excellence series produced by the National League for Nursing, this resource provides general recommendations for communicating with people with a variety of disabilities.

- **Disability Rights Education & Defense Fund (DREDF): Healthcare Stories (https://dredf.org/healthcare-stories/index/):** This series of videos shares real-life stories told by people with disability as they have made efforts to obtain quality healthcare. People with a variety of disabilities are included.

- **The NYS Health Foundation: A Blueprint for Improving Access to Primary Care for Adults with Physical Disabilities (https://nyshealthfoundation.org/resource/blueprint-for-improving-access-to-primary-care-adults-physical-disabilities/):** This blueprint was created by the Independence Care System (ICS) to improve primary care for adults with physical disability. The blueprint contains useful information for healthcare professionals and for individuals with disability.

- **Ohio Disability and Health Program/Disability Healthcare Training (https://nisonger.osu.edu/education-training/ohio-disability-health-program/disability-healthcare-training/):** This online training resource is designed to increase healthcare providers' competence in caring for those with physical/sensory and developmental disabilities and addresses healthcare access for people with disabilities. These two 1-hour sessions are approved for continuing education by the Centers for Disease Control and Prevention for physicians, nurses, certified health education specialists, and other health professionals.

- **Professor Tom Shakespeare: Disability as Identity (https://youtu.be/QMPb_554c5o or https://www.youtube.com/watch?v=QMPb_554c5o):** This is a video of Professor Tom Shakespeare speaking at the Manchester Division of Clinical Psychology's 2019 conference. Professor Shakespeare writes, talks, and conducts research about disability as well as about ethical issues related to prenatal genetic testing and end-of-life issues.

- **Professor Tom Shakespeare: Disability: Better Understood as a Public Health or Human Rights Issue? (https://vimeo.com/321259239):** In this video, Professor Tom Shakespeare explores how best to approach the issue of disability.

- **Susan M. Havercamp, PhD, Kenneth Robey, PhD, and Suzanne Smeltzer, EdD, RN, FAAN: Approaches to Training Healthcare Providers on Working with Patients with Disabilities (https://fndusa.org/wp-content/uploads/2015/05/Approaches-to-Training-Healthcare-Providers.pdf):** This resource provides a set of slides with approaches to teach healthcare students and professionals about disability. Sponsored by the Association of University Centers on Disability (AUCD) and the Alliance for Disability in Health Care Education (ADHCE).

- **Villanova University M. Louise Fitzpatrick College of Nursing: Caring for People with Disabilities: The Nurse Practitioner Tool Kit (https://www1.villanova.edu/villanova/nursing/community/npsknowdisabilitycare.html):** This resource includes information, teaching materials, videos, and other materials necessary for nursing faculty to prepare nurse practitioner students and graduates to care for people with disability.

SUMMARY

Although physical disability is the most visible type of disability, people with physical disability continue to encounter barriers that limit their ability to receive quality healthcare. Healthcare professionals and others often harbor negative attitudes toward people with physical disability and may fail to make accommodations that would enable them to receive quality care. Improving attitudes of healthcare providers would go a long way toward improving care for people with physical disability but is inadequate if healthcare providers are not knowledgeable about the implications of having a physical disability with respect to healthcare. This chapter provided an overview of the consequences of physical disability and suggested strategies to improve care for this population. Several examples of physical disability were discussed and aspects of care for patients with physical disability across settings were presented. Finally, the chapter identified resources to learn more about physical disability and to teach others about it, and to consider the implications for providing care of individuals with physical disability.

REFERENCES

American Diabetes Association. (2020a). 1. Improving care and promoting health in populations: Standards of medical care in diabetes—2020. *Diabetes Care, 43*(Suppl. 1), S7–S13. doi:10.2337/dc20-S001

American Diabetes Association. (2020b). 10. Cardiovascular disease and risk management: Standards of medical care in diabetes—2020. *Diabetes Care, 43*(Suppl. 1), S111–S134. doi:10.2337/dc20-S010

American Diabetes Association. (2020c). 11. Microvascular complications and foot care: Standards of medical care in diabetes—2020. *Diabetes Care, 43*(Suppl. 1), S135–S151. doi:10.2337/dc19-S011

Centers for Disease Control and Prevention. (n.d.-a). Common barriers to participation experienced by people with disabilities. Retrieved from https://www.cdc.gov/ncbddd/disabilityandhealth/disability-barriers.html

Centers for Disease Control and Prevention. (n.d.-b). Disability and health overview. Retrieved from https://www.cdc.gov/ncbddd/disabilityandhealth/documents/disabilities_impacts_all_of_us.pdf

Centers for Disease Control and Prevention. (n.d.-c). Disability and health related conditions. Retrieved from https://www.cdc.gov/ncbddd/disabilityandhealth/relatedconditions.html

Centers for Disease Control and Prevention. (n.d.-d). National diabetes statistics report, 2020. Retrieved from https://www.cdc.gov/diabetes/library/features/diabetes-stat-report.html

Centers for Disease Control and Prevention. (n.d.-e). National Health Interview Survey (NHIS) public use data release. Retrieved from ftp://ftp.cdc.gov/pub/Health_Statistics/NCHS/Dataset_Documentation/NHIS/2016/srvydesc.pdf

Centers for Disease Control and Prevention. (n.d.-f). TBI data and statistics. Retrieved from https://www.cdc.gov/traumaticbraininjury/data/index.html

Dokken, B. B. (2008). The pathophysiology of cardiovascular disease and diabetes: Beyond blood pressure and lipids. *Diabetes Spectrum, 21*(3), 160–165. doi:10.2337/diaspect.21.3.160

Forman-Hoffman, V. L., Ault, K. L., Anderson, W. L., Weiner, J. M., Stevens, A., Campbell, V. A., & Armour, B. S. (2015). Disability status, mortality, and leading causes of death in the United States community population. *Medical Care, 53*(4), 346–354. doi:10.1097/MLR.0000000000000321

Ghasemi, N., Razavi, S., & Nikzad, E. (2017). Multiple sclerosis: Pathogenesis, symptoms, diagnoses and cell-based therapy. *Cell Journal, 19*(1), 1–10. doi:10.22074/cellj.2016.4867

Global Burden of Disease 2017 Disease and Injury Incidence and Prevalence Collaborators. (2018). Global, regional, and national incidence, prevalence, and years lived with disability for 354 diseases and injuries for 195 countries and territories, 1990–2017: A systematic analysis for the Global Burden of Disease Study 2017. *The Lancet, 392*(10159), P1789–P1858. doi:10.1016/S0140-6736(18)32279-7

Independence Care System. (2016). A blueprint for improving access to primary care for adults with physical disabilities. Retrieved from https://nyshealthfoundation.org/wp-content/uploads/2017/12/A_Blueprint_for_Improving_Access_to_Primary_Care_for_Adults_with_Physical_Disabilities.pdf

Long-Bellil, L., Mitra, M., Iezzoni, L. I., Smeltzer, S. C., & Smith, L. D. (2017). Experiences and unmet needs of women with physical disabilities for pain relief during labor and delivery. *Disability and Health Journal, 10*(3), 440–444. doi:10.1016/j.dhjo.2017.02.007

McCarthy, E. P., Ngo, L. H., Roetzheim, R. G., Chirikos, T. N., Li, D., Drews, R. E., & Iezzoni, L. I. (2006). Disparities in breast cancer treatment and survival for women with disabilities. *Annals of Internal Medicine, 145*(9), 637–645.

Mitra, M., Long-Bellil, L. M., Iezzoni, L I., Smeltzer, S. C., & Smith, L. D. (2016). Pregnancy among women with physical disabilities: Unmet needs and recommendations on navigating pregnancy. *Disability and Health Journal, 9*(3), 457–463. doi:10.1016/j.dhjo.2015.12.007

National Council on Disability. (2015). Transportation update: Where we've gone and what we've learned. Retrieved from https://ncd.gov/publications/2015/05042015/

National Institute of Neurological Disorders and Stroke. (2019). Spina bifida fact sheet. Retrieved from https://www.ninds.nih.gov/Disorders/Patient-Caregiver-Education/Fact-Sheets/Spina-Bifida-Fact-Sheet

National Spinal Cord Injury Statistical Center. (2018). Spinal cord injury facts and figures at a glance. Retrieved from https://www.nscisc.uab.edu/Public/Facts%20and%20Figures%20-%202018.pdf

Okoro, C. A., Hollis, N. D., Cyrus, A. C., & Griffin-Blake, S. (2018). Prevalence of disabilities and health care access by disability status and type among adults—United States, 2016. *Morbidity and Mortality Weekly Report, 67*(32), 882–887. doi: 10.15585/mmwr.mm6732a3

Reichard, A., Stolzle, H., & Fox, M. H. (2011). Health disparities among adults with physical disabilities or cognitive limitations compared to individuals with no disabilities in the United States. *Disability and Health Journal, 4*(2), 59–67. doi:10.1016/j.dhjo.2010.05.003

Satchidanand, N., Gunukula, S. K., Lam, W. Y., McGuigan, D., New, I., Symons, A. B., ... Akl, E. A. (2012). Attitudes of healthcare students and professionals toward patients with physical disability: A systematic review. *American Journal of Physical Medicine and Rehabilitation, 91*(6), 533–545. doi:10.1097/PHM.0b013e3182555ea4

Shulman, L. M. (2010). Understanding disability in Parkinson's disease. *Movement Disorders, 25*(Suppl 1), S131–S135. doi:10.1002/mds.22789

Sinclair, L. B., Taft, K. E., Sloan, M. L., Stevens, A. C., & Krahn, G. L. (2015). Tools for improving clinical preventive services receipt among women with disabilities of childbearing ages and beyond. *Maternal and Child Health Journal. 19*(6), 1,189–1,201. doi:10.1007/s10995-014-1627-4

Smeltzer, S. C., Avery, C., & Haynor, P. (2012). Interactions of people with disabilities with nursing staff during hospitalization. *American Journal of Nursing, 112*(4), 30–37. doi:10.1097/01.NAJ.0000413454.07369.e3

Smeltzer, S. C., Mariani, B., Ross, J., de Mange, P., Meakim, C., Bruderle, E., & Nthenge, S. (2015). Persons with disability: Their experiences as standardized patients in an undergraduate nursing program. *Nursing Education Perspectives, 36*(6), 398–400. doi:10.5480/15-1592

Smeltzer, S. C., Mitra, M., Iezzoni, L. I., Long-Bellil, L., & Smith, L. D. (2016). Perinatal experiences of women with physical disabilities and their recommendations for clinicians. *Journal of Obstetric, Gynecologic, and Neonatal Nursing, 45*(6), 781–789. doi: 10.1016/j.jogn.2016.07.007

Smeltzer, S. C., Ross, J. G., Mariani, B., Meakim, C. H., Bruderle, E., de Mange, E., & Nthenge, S. (2018). Innovative approach to address disability concepts and standardized patients with disability in an undergraduate curriculum. *Journal of Nursing Education, 57*(12), 760–764. doi:10.3928/01484834-20181119-11

Smeltzer, S. C., Wint, A. J., Ecker, J. L., & Iezzoni, L. I. (2017). Labor, delivery and anesthesia experiences of women with physical disability. *Birth, 44*(4), 315–324. doi: 10.1111/birt.12296

United States Bone and Joint Initiative. (2016). The impact of musculoskeletal disorders on Americans—Opportunities for action. Retrieved from https://www.boneandjointburden.org/docs/BMUSExecutiveSummary2016.pdf

US Census Bureau. (2014). Survey of income and program participation. Retrieved from https://www.census.gov/sipp/

World Health Organization. (2011). World report on disability. Retrieved from https://www.who.int/publications/i/item/world-report-on-disability

World Health Organization. (2015). WHO global disability action plan 2014–2021. Retrieved from https://apps.who.int/iris/bitstream/handle/10665/199544/9789241509619_eng.pdf;jsessionid=AADCCC322C621CDC2BDBA238C05A28D6?sequence=1

World Health Organization. (2018). Disability and health. Retrieved from https://www.who.int/news-room/fact-sheets/detail/disability-and-health

World Health Organization. (2019). Musculoskeletal conditions. Retrieved from https://www.who.int/news-room/fact-sheets/detail/musculoskeletal-conditions

Wu, X., Li, Z., Cao, J., Jiao, J., Wang, Y., Liu, G., ... Wan, X. (2018). The association between major complications of immobility during hospitalization and quality of life among bedridden patients: A 3 month prospective multi-center study. *PLoS One, 13*(10), e0205729. doi:10.1371/journal.pone.0205729

Ziegler, Graham, K., MacKenzie, E. J., Ephraim, P. L., Travison, T. G., & Brookmeyer, R. (2008). Estimating the prevalence of limb loss in the United States: 2005 to 2050. *Archives of Physical Medicine and Rehabilitation, 89*(3), 422–429. doi:10.1016/j.apmr.2007.11.005

6

PSYCHIATRIC/MENTAL HEALTH DISABILITY AND NEUROCOGNITIVE DISORDERS

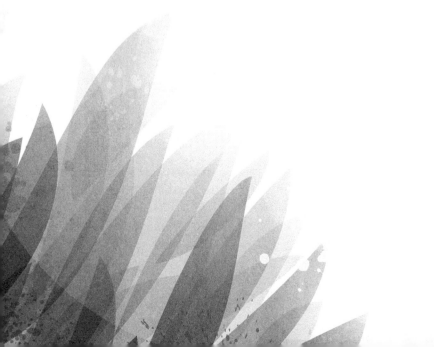

INTRODUCTION

The term *psychiatric/mental health* (PMH) disability describes a wide range of mental and emotional conditions. Psychiatric/mental health disorders are common in the US. However, not all these disorders result in or qualify as a mental disability, as defined by the Americans with Disabilities Act (ADA) of 1990 and the ADA Amendments Act (ADAAA) of 2008 (P.L. 110-325). This definition is as follows:

> Mental disability refers to a mental impairment that substantially limits one or more major life activities of an individual; having a record of such an impairment; or being regarded as having such as impairment.

The term *psychiatric/mental disability* describes only part of the ADA's broader term of *mental impairment* (National Rehabilitation Information Center, 2014). Mental disability or mental impairment as addressed by the ADA also includes:

- Learning disability
- Developmental disability
- Intellectual disability
- Neurocognitive disability
- Disability resulting from brain injury

These are discussed in Chapter 4 and Chapter 5.

Psychiatric/mental disability—discussed in this chapter—refers to a PMH illness that significantly interferes with a person's ability to engage in major life activities such as learning, working, and communicating.

There is less written about psychiatric disability than about other disabilities or PMH disorders (Rudnick, 2014). However, policy guidance from the Equal Employment Opportunity Commission

(EEOC, 2002) addresses many questions about psychiatric disability in the context of the ADA. Although the EEOC's main focus is on employment issues as they relate to disability (including psychiatric disability), its guidance is helpful for understanding psychiatric/mental disability.

According to the EEOC, the ADA's definition of mental impairment includes any mental or psychological disorders such as emotional or mental illness. These include the following examples:

- Major depression

- Bipolar disorder

- Anxiety disorders (including panic disorder, obsessive compulsive disorder, and post-traumatic stress disorder)

- Schizophrenia

- Personality disorders

The EEOC (2002) guidance also lists major life activities relevant to psychiatric disability. These are as follows:

- Thinking

- Concentrating

- Interacting with others

- Caring for oneself

- Speaking

- Performing manual tasks

- Working

The American Psychiatric Association's (APA) 2015 *Diagnostic and Statistical Manual of Mental Disorders* (DSM-5) is the key reference on PMH disorders for mental health professionals for the purposes of diagnosis and insurance reimbursement. However, not all disorders included in *DSM-5* are considered disabilities or impairments. According to the ADA, for an impairment to be considered a disability, its effect on a person's major life activities must be significant. When a PMH disorder is severe enough to prevent a person from performing such activities—or significantly restricts the condition, manner, or duration under which the person can perform compared to the average person in the general population (EEOC, 2002)—it is considered a disability. Determining whether a limitation is a "substantial limitation" depends on its severity and on the length of time it restricts major life activities.

There are many mental health conditions or disorders. They vary in severity from mild to moderate to severe. Two broad categories of mental health conditions identified by the National Institute of Mental Health (NIMH, 2019) are:

- **Any mental illness (AMI):** This includes all types of mental illnesses.

- **Serious mental illness (SMI):** This is a mental, behavioral, or emotional disorder resulting in serious functional impairment that interferes with or limits one or more major life activities, thus meeting the definition of mental disability.

NIMH (2019) states that the burden of mental illness is particularly concentrated among people with SMI. Because of the high prevalence rates, few US families are untouched by mental illness.

Zimmerman, Morgan, and Stanton (2018) observe that the severity of PMH disorders is difficult to determine. This is because of the various ways in which *severity* can be defined:

- Frequency of symptoms

- Number of symptoms

- Intensity of symptoms

- Impact of symptoms on function or quality of life

The severity of symptoms influences decisions about level and type of care as well as decisions to seek support due to PMH disability.

Other terminology that captures the meaning of PMH disability includes the following:

- Persistent psychiatric disability

- Severe and persistent mental illness

- Severe, persistent psychiatric disability

Other terms used to describe PMH disorders include *behavioral and emotional disorders* and *pervasive developmental disorders*. Their severity and effects on life activities determine if these disorders are considered PMH disability.

Although neurocognitive disorder (formerly and commonly referred to as *dementia*) is not a PMH disorder, illness, or disability, it is discussed in this chapter because it shares many characteristics with a number of PMH disorders and disabilities. In its DSM-5 (2015), the APA defines major *neurocognitive disorders* as disorders with significant cognitive decline in one or more of the following neurocognitive domains:

- Complex attention

- Executive function

- Learning

- Memory

- Language

- Perceptual-motor function

- Social cognition

The extensive lists of PMH disorders in the APA *DSM-5* (2015) and in the *World Health Organization (WHO) ICD-11 Classification of Mental and Behavioral Disorders, Clinical Descriptions and Diagnostic Guideline* (2018a) attest to the complexity and variation in PMH disorders and disability.

Social cognition refers to one's ability to inhibit unwanted behavior, recognize social cues, read facial expressions, express empathy, motivate oneself, alter behavior in response to feedback, and develop insight (Sachdev et al., 2014).

Neurocognitive disorder is now considered the correct term to describe this condition. One reason for the change in terminology is the stigma associated with the term *dementia* (Sachdev et al., 2014). However, the lay public and many professional organizations will likely continue to use *dementia*.

To be considered a major neurocognitive disorder, cognitive deficits must interfere with one's independence and daily life such that assistance is needed with instrumental activities of daily living. (This is consistent with the ADA's definition of disability.)

PREVALENCE OF PSYCHIATRIC/MENTAL HEALTH DISABILITY

According to the NIMH (2019), nearly 47.6 million adults in the US—1 in every 5 adults—live with a mental illness. NIMH estimates that 22.1% of US adults over the age of 18 have a mental disorder or disability. Psychological, behavioral, and psychiatric disabilities account for 4 of the 10 leading causes of disability (NIMH, 2019). One in 25 US adults experiences serious mental illness (SMI) as defined earlier in this chapter.

The prevalence of any mental illness (AMI) differs among ethnic groups (National Association of Mental Illness [NAMI], 2018):

- 20.4% of non-Hispanic white adults

- 16% of non-Hispanic Black or African American adults

- 15% of non-Hispanic Asian adults

- 17% of Hispanic or Latinx adults

- 27% of adults who report mixed/multiracial

In addition, AMI affects 37.4% of lesbian, gay, and bisexual adults.

According to NIMH (2019), an estimated 11.4 million (4.5%) adults age 18 or older in the US had serious mental illness (SMI) in 2018. Of these, 7.5 million (66.7%) had received mental health treatment within the previous year, but 35.9%—more than one-third—had not. Lack of health insurance and access to an appropriate mental health care provider contributed to lack of treatment.

The prevalence rates of the more common types of PMH disorders that can result in disability in US adults are as follows (NIMH, 2018):

- **Major depressive episode:** 7.2% (estimated 17.7 million people)

- **Schizophrenia:** <1% (estimated 1.5 million people)

- **Bipolar disorder:** 2.8% (estimated 7 million people)

- **Anxiety disorders:** 19.1% (estimated 48 million people)

- **Post-traumatic stress disorder:** 3.6% (estimated 9 million people)

- **Obsessive compulsive disorder:** 1.2% (estimated 3 million people)

- **Borderline personality disorder:** 1.4% (estimated 3.5 million people)

SUMMARY OF PREVALENCE AND TREATMENT RATES OF PEOPLE WITH MENTAL ILLNESS

- Nearly 1 in every 5 adults (47.6 million, or 19.1% of US adults) has any mental illness (AMI).
- One in every 25 US adults (11.4 million people) experiences serious mental illness (SMI) each year, which represents 1 in every 4 US adults with mental illness.
- The prevalence of SMI is higher among women (5.7%) than men (3.3%).
- Young adults age 18 to 25 years have the highest prevalence of SMI (7.7%). This is compared to adults age 26 to 49 years (5.9%) and those 50 years of age and older (2.5%).
- One in every 6 (7.7 million) US youth experiences a mental health disorder each year. 50% of lifetime mental illness begins by 14 years of age and 75% by age 24.
- The average delay between onset of mental illness symptoms and treatment is 11 years.

- The percentage of young adults (18–25 years old) with SMI who received mental health treatment (57.4%) was lower than adults with SMI age 26 to 49 years (66.2%) and age 50 and older (75.6%).
- Those with SMI who received no treatment included 46.2% of young adults with SMI and 36.3% of adults 26 to 49 years of age with SMI.
- More women with SMI (71.5%) received treatment than men with SMI (57.7%).

(McCance-Katz, 2019)

PREVALENCE OF NEUROCOGNITIVE DISORDERS

The World Health Organization (WHO) has declared neurocognitive disorders a public health priority and a global epidemic. More than 50 million people around the world have neurocognitive disorders, with nearly 10 million new cases each year (WHO, 2015). It is estimated that there will be almost 76 million cases in 2030 and more than 135 million cases by 2050.

Dementia due to Alzheimer's disease (AD) is the most common form of neurocognitive disorder. It may contribute 60% to 70% of cases globally, making it one of the major causes of disability and dependency among older people. In the US, approximately 5.7 million people are living with neurocognitive disorders (Alzheimer's Association, 2018; Plassman et al., 2007). Alzheimer's disease accounts for approximately 60% to 70% of these cases, followed by vascular dementia and other causes (National Institute on Aging [NIA], 2019; WHO, 2017a). As with global trends, these numbers are expected to rise as life expectancy increases. It is estimated that the total number of people living with dementia due to Alzheimer's disease in the US will be 13.8 million by 2050. More women have Alzheimer's or other neurocognitive disorders than men, with almost two-thirds of those with Alzheimer's dementia being women.

CAUSES OF PSYCHIATRIC/MENTAL HEALTH DISABILITY

Although no single cause of mental health disorders has been identified, multiple theories exist as to the causes of PMH disorders and disability.

Factors recognized as possible contributors to mental health disorders include the following:

- Genetics

- Environment

- Lifestyle/social factors and their interaction

Biochemical processes and changes in basic brain structure have also been identified as having a role. For example, it has been suggested that changes in neurotransmitters in the brain—such as serotonin, dopamine, glutamate, and norepinephrine—play an important role in depression and schizophrenia (NAMI, 2018; National Institutes of Health [NIH], 2007; WHO, 2019).

Changes in brain chemistry resulting from substance abuse have also been identified as a factor. Substance use disorder occurs in a substantial portion of the population of people with mental illness. In 2016, nearly 45 million adults were reported to have a mental disorder alone, 11 million had a substance use disorder alone, and 8 million had both a mental disorder and a substance use disorder (NAMI, 2018; NIH, 2007; Owens, Fingar, McDermott, Muhri, & Heslin, 2019; WHO, 2019).

Environmental factors have also been identified as increasing risk of mental health illness. These factors include the following:

- Head or brain injury

- Poor nutrition

- Exposure to environmental toxins (e.g., lead or cigarette smoke)

- A stressful environment in the home or work setting
- Traumatic life events such as being the victim of a crime or violence

Still, a single event or situation is unlikely to trigger the onset of PMH disorders or disability.

The combination of genetic, environmental, and social factors has been implicated in determining whether one's mental illness is mild or severe. Several specific types of mental illness are more likely if there is a family history of mental illness. PMH disorders more likely to have a genetic component include the following (Centers for Disease Control and Prevention [CDC)] 2012; NIH, 2007; WHO, 2019):

- Autism or autism spectrum disorder (ASD)
- Bipolar disorder
- Schizophrenia
- Attention-deficit/hyperactivity disorder (ADHD)

The CDC (2012) identified the following as risk factors for PMH disorders:

- Family history
- Stressful life conditions
- Having a chronic disease
- Traumatic experiences
- Use of illegal drugs
- Childhood abuse or neglect
- Lack of social support

The CDC (2012) describes PMH disorders as medical conditions that disrupt a person's thinking, feeling, mood, ability to relate to others, and daily functioning. The CDC notes that mental health disorders are treatable and that those with serious mental illnesses can obtain relief with an appropriate treatment plan. According to the NIH (2007), although PMH disorders cannot be cured, they can often be treated effectively to minimize the symptoms and allow those affected persons to function in work, school, or social environments. However, as indicated, a sizable percentage of those with PMH illnesses do not receive needed treatment.

CAUSES OF NEUROCOGNITIVE DISORDERS

Neurocognitive disorders occur as a result of damage or destruction of nerve cells in parts of the brain involved in cognitive function. With dementia due to Alzheimer's disease—the most common variety of neurocognitive disorder—progressive accumulation of the protein fragment beta-amyloid (plaques) appears in the brain, along with inflammation and atrophy of cells of the brain.

Genetic mutations are thought to be responsible in many cases of neurocognitive disorders. In addition, risk factors for vascular dementia include the following (WHO, 2017b):

- Low level of education
- Hypertension
- Diabetes
- Obesity
- Smoking
- Metabolic syndrome

These factors also increase the risk of Alzheimer's disease.

Another cause of neurocognitive disorder is *traumatic brain injury* (TBI), including so-called "mild" TBI, in which repeated trauma to the brain has resulted in concussion. Other disorders with which dementia may present include (but are not limited to) the following (Alzheimer's Association, 2018):

- HIV infection
- Huntington's disease
- Lewy body disease
- Parkinson's disease
- Prion disease
- Substance and/or medication use

There is some evidence that nutritious diet, physical activity, social engagement, and mentally stimulating pursuits may reduce the risk of neurocognitive disorders and help older people to remain healthy as they age (NIA, 2019).

CONSEQUENCES OF PSYCHIATRIC/ MENTAL HEALTH DISABILITY

A startling and important consequence of PMH illness and disability is the significantly higher mortality rate among people with mental health disorders than comparison populations (Walker, McGee, & Druss, 2015). WHO (2018b) estimates that those with severe mental disorders have a 2 to 3 times higher average mortality than the general population. This translates to a reduction in life expectancy by 10 to 20 years.

An analysis of multiple studies shows that 67.3% of deaths among people with PMH disorders were due to natural causes, 17.5% to unnatural causes (e.g., suicide and unintentional injuries), and the remainder to other or unknown causes. Walker et al. (2015) estimate that 14.3% of deaths worldwide—or approximately 8 million deaths each year—are due to PMH disorders. Walker et al. (2015) also identify high rates of tobacco smoking, substance use, physical inactivity, and poor diet as common in people with PMH disorders. These factors contribute to the high rates of chronic medical conditions among them.

Prevention and care of chronic medical conditions among people with PMH disorders require promotion of healthy behaviors, early diagnosis, and care related to multiple conditions (Walker et al., 2015), similar to care for individuals without PMH. However, people with PMH disorders generally receive less in the way of information related to health promotion in addition to receiving inadequate general and preventive healthcare (e.g., immunizations, cancer screening, or smoking cessation counseling and assistance).

> The mortality gap between people with schizophrenia and the general population has been increasing over time. However, a shorter life span pertains to people with a variety of mental illness disorders, not just schizophrenia.

The CDC (2012) identified complications of untreated PMH disorders as the primary cause of missed work and lack of participation when at work. Previous experiences with or fear of social stigma and discrimination often prevent people with PMH disorders who need treatment from acknowledging their mental health issues and obtaining appropriate medical care (CDC, 2012).

In a recent study of annual health spending for medical conditions, PMH disorders topped the list of most costly conditions, with annual spending at $201 billion. This amount exceeded that of all other medical conditions, including cardiac disease, trauma, and cancer (Roehrig, 2016).

NAMI (2018) has described the ripple effect of PMH disorders by summarizing their impact on the person, family, community, and world at large. These include the following:

- **Individual level:** Impacts on the individual level include increased risk for chronic disease (e.g., diabetes or cancer), higher rate of cardiovascular and metabolic disease (twice as high in adults with SMI), unemployment, and high school dropout rate (NAMI, 2018).

- **Family level:** Impacts on the family level include require-ments for increased caregiving by families. At least 8.4 mil-lion Americans provide care to an adult with an emotional or mental illness or substance abuse problem. Caregivers spend an average of 32 hours per week providing unpaid care for family members with mental illness (NAMI, 2018).

- **Community level:** At the community level, mental and substance use disorders result in high incidence of emer-gency department visits (1 in 8, or 12 million visits). Mood disorders are the most common cause of hospitalization (other than childbirth) for all people in the US under age 45. In the US, 20% of people who are homeless have a serious mental illness, as do 37% of people incarcerated in state and federal prison and 16.5% of youth offenders. Costs associated with serious mental illness include $193.2 billion in lost earnings across the US economy each year (NAMI, 2018).

- **Global level:** Depression and anxiety disorders alone cost the global economy $1 trillion each year in lost productiv-ity, with depression identified as the leading cause of dis-ability worldwide (NAMI, 2018).

Increased risk of suicide also affects people with PMH disor-ders and disability, their families, and communities at large. NAMI (2018) reports that 46% of people who die by suicide had a diag-nosed mental health disorder and 90% displayed or reported symp-toms of PMH disorder (based on interviews with family, friends, and healthcare professionals). Suicide is the second leading cause of death among people between 10 and 34 years of age and the tenth leading cause of death in the US overall. Of particular concern is NAMI's (2018) report that the overall suicide rate in the US in-creased by 31% since 2001. The incidence of suicide is much higher in men than women, with 75% of suicide cases being males.

A major issue is the stigma associated with PMH illness and disability and dementia (neurocognitive disorder). It has been described as the last great stigma of the twentieth century. Not only are negative and derogatory words often used to describe people with these disorders, but often those affected are blamed for their PMH disability or neurocognitive disorder and are considered irresponsible, childlike, and even dangerous (NIH, 2007). The reality is that most people with PMH disorders can take care of themselves and carry on with their lives despite their illness, including working, attending school, and living independently.

> Despite these numbers, it's important to note that most people with PMH disorders do not commit suicide. The risk of suicide is estimated to be 5 to 8% for several PMH disorders—mainly depression, alcoholism, and schizophrenia (Brådvik, 2018).

Misconceptions about people with PMH illness and disability are based on inaccurate and false information. Stigma and negative attitudes toward those with these disorders can and do occur in healthcare and among healthcare professionals. This can have devastating effects if those with PMH illness and disability avoid healthcare and treatment that could be helpful. In a recent review of literature on nurses' perceptions and beliefs about people with PMH disorders, Ross and Goldner (2009) reported that some nurses had negative attitudes, prejudices, and fears due to stereotypical beliefs that people with these disorders are unpredictable, violent, bizarre, and even dangerous, even though these stereotypes are incorrect. Some nurses incorrectly interpret distress on the part of those with these disorders as a symptom of mental illness and are concerned that saying or doing the wrong thing could result in them reacting with uncontrollable behavior. Because of these misconceptions and stereotyping, people with PMH disorders and their families have reported being treated in a demeaning and noncaring way by nurses in general medical-surgical and emergency department settings. Consequences include fragmentation of care and the devaluation of patients and their psychiatric/mental health care needs.

> Lack of knowledge and lack of interaction with people with psychiatric/mental health illness and disability are factors in nurses' stereotyping and negative attitudes.

CONSEQUENCES OF NEUROCOGNITIVE DISORDERS

Neurocognitive disorders cause impaired cognitive function that results in an inability to carry out decision-making and other usual activities of daily living. They also damage other parts of the brain, eventually resulting in the inability to carry out usual physical activities, including walking, communicating, and swallowing, and eventual death (Alzheimer's Association, 2018).

Although older people are often able to cope well with physical changes that occur with aging, and even remain fairly independent, those with the cognitive impairment that characterizes neurocognitive disorders are often unable to adjust to changes. Their ability to carry out complex tasks and eventually even simple, routine activities becomes impaired. They also have difficulty meeting their basic personal care hygiene needs (WHO, 2017a).

Impaired communication is a major issue for people with neurocognitive disorders, eventually affecting most aspects of their lives. In the early stages of a neurocognitive disorder, those affected are usually able to understand, participate in, and contribute to conversation—although excessive noise and other stimulation may make it difficult for them to follow along. As neurocognitive disorders progress, however, those affected are unlikely to remember names of family and friends, places, objects, and what was just said to them. They may talk about the past, have increasing difficulty finding words, repeat themselves (asking the same questions and telling the same stories), and drift in conversation from one topic to another. In the late stages of neurocognitive disorders, the person may be unable to communicate verbally or in writing and may rely only on gestures (Alzheimer's Association, 2018). Nonverbal behaviors such as agitation, restlessness, and combativeness often become the only way people with neurocognitive disorders can express themselves and their needs (Zembrzuski, 2019).

As with psychiatric/mental health disorders, people with neurocognitive disorders require a tremendous amount of care. People with Alzheimer's disease receive more than 18.5 billion hours of informal care each year, usually from family members—equivalent to $234 billion (Alzheimer's Association, 2018).

If suicide occurs with a neurocognitive disorder, it is more likely to happen in the early phases of cognitive decline (Conejero et al., 2018). Among veterans, those who are younger, and often those who have new diagnoses of neurocognitive disorder, are more likely to commit suicide. People with psychiatric symptoms of depression and anxiety who are early in the course of a neurocognitive disorder are at greatest risk for suicide (Seyfried, Kales, Ignacio, Conwell, & Valenstein, 2011).

Just as stigma occurs with PMH disability, it also occurs with neurocognitive disorders. Stigma associated with neurocognitive disorders is widespread and has a profound effect on those with neurocognitive disorders and their families. They are often isolated or even hidden away because of fears about negative reactions from friends, neighbors, and relatives. Stigma can result in delays in seeking diagnosis and treatment and can have negative effects on relationships with others, including healthcare professionals. People with neurocognitive disorders report feeling marginalized and their views and opinions discounted. Instead of remaining engaged in family and community activities, people with neurocognitive disorders and their families may disengage because of stigma. This further isolates them from others and from activities that could contribute to their well-being (CDC, 2015).

CHARACTERISTICS OF SELECT PSYCHIATRIC/MENTAL HEALTH DISABILITIES

As stated, there are many different categories and types of PMH disabilities. Table 6.1 contains details on some specific types of PMH disabilities. This list is not intended to be exhaustive.

TABLE 6.1   DESCRIPTIONS AND CHARACTERISTICS OF SELECT PSYCHIATRIC/MENTAL HEALTH DISABILITIES

GENERAL DESCRIPTION	COMMON FEATURES OR CHARACTERISTICS
MAJOR DEPRESSIVE EPISODE	
A common but serious mood disorder. There are several forms of depression: • **Persistent depressive disorder:** This lasts for at least two years. With this form of depression, the person may have episodes of major depression along with periods of less severe symptoms. • **Postpartum depression:** This is full-blown major depression during pregnancy or after delivery. It is characterized by extreme sadness, anxiety, and exhaustion, making it difficult for new mothers to engage in daily care activities for themselves or their babies. • **Psychotic depression:** This describes severe depression plus some form of psychosis, such as delusions or hallucinations. • **Seasonal affective disorder:** This is characterized by the onset of depression during the winter months, when there is less natural sunlight, that generally lifts during spring and summer. It predictably returns every year. To be diagnosed with depression, symptoms must be present for at least two weeks. Depression occurs in 7.2% of the population and 9.5% of those with PMH disorders.	• Affects how one feels, thinks, and handles daily activities, such as sleeping, eating, or working • Typically accompanied by social withdrawal, increased sleep, and weight gain

SCHIZOPHRENIA

Chronic, severe mental disorder that affects how a person thinks, feels, and behaves. Those affected may seem like they have lost touch with reality. Schizophrenia is not as common as other mental disorders, but it is very disabling. It occurs in less than 1% of US adults (2.4 million adults), but the consequences can be profound. Age at onset is typically late teens to early 20s for men, and late 20s to early 30s for women.

Factors implicated as causes include genetics, environment, changes in brain chemistry, and substance use.

There are four categories of symptoms:

- **Positive symptoms:** Psychotic behaviors not generally seen in healthy people, such as losing touch with some aspects of reality, hallucinations, delusions, thought disorders, movement disorders (agitated body movements)

- **Negative symptoms:** Disruptions of normal emotions and behaviors, flat affect, reduced feelings of pleasure in everyday life, difficulty beginning and sustaining activities, reduced speaking

- **Cognitive symptoms:** Subtle or severe changes in memory or other aspects of thinking, poor executive functioning, difficulty focusing or paying attention, poor working memory (the ability to use information immediately after learning it)

- **Affective symptoms:** Involving emotions and their expression

continues

TABLE 6.1 DESCRIPTIONS AND CHARACTERISTICS OF SELECT PSYCHIATRIC/MENTAL HEALTH DISABILITIES (CONT.)

GENERAL DESCRIPTION	COMMON FEATURES OR CHARACTERISTICS
BIPOLAR DISORDER	
Disorder in which the affected person experiences episodes of extreme low moods that meet the criteria for major depression (*bipolar depression*) and episodes of extreme high moods—euphoric or irritable (*mania* or *hypomania*). It is estimated to affect 2.8% of the adult population, or 7 million people.	• Extreme mood swings • Extreme highs and very low lows
ANXIETY DISORDER	
Disorder characterized by persistent feelings ranging from apprehension or uneasiness to overwhelming alarm or terror. Anxiety disorder affects 18% of adults with psychiatric/mental health disorders.	• Persistent feelings of apprehension or uneasiness • Overwhelming feelings of alarm or terror that can occur with ordinary, everyday events • Recurring nightmares • Painful, intrusive memories
OBSESSIVE COMPULSIVE DISORDER	
Repetitive or ritualistic behavior employed to reduce or control symptoms of anxiety such as recurrent thoughts or impulses, recurring nightmares, or painful intrusive memories. Obsessive compulsive disorder (OCD) affects 1.2% of the US adult population, or an estimated 3 million people.	• Repetitive or ritualistic behavior employed to reduce or control symptoms of anxiety

CHARACTERISTICS OF SELECT NEUROCOGNITIVE DISORDERS

As with examples of PMH disorders, there are numerous neurocognitive disorders. (See Table 6.2.) Examples provided illustrate common types of neurocognitive disorders.

TABLE 6.2   DESCRIPTIONS AND CHARACTERISTICS OF SELECT NEUROCOGNITIVE DISORDERS

GENERAL DESCRIPTION	COMMON FEATURES OR CHARACTERISTICS
ALZHEIMER'S DISEASE (AD) DEMENTIA	
A degenerative brain disease. AD is the most common type of dementia, accounting for 60 to 80% of cases. Incidence of AD increases with age. Common causes of AD include the progressive accumulation of protein fragment beta-amyloid (plaques) in the brain and genetic mutations. The disease is common in people with Down syndrome.	• **Early symptoms:** Difficulty remembering names, events, or recent conversations; apathy and depression; difficulty completing familiar tasks • **Late symptoms:** Impaired judgment and decision-making ability; inability to plan or organize; impaired communication; disorientation and confusion; inability to swallow or walk
VASCULAR DEMENTIA	
Caused by impaired vascular supply to the brain, vascular dementia accounts for about 5 to 10% of dementia cases. It may contribute to symptoms of AD and can occur with other types of neurocognitive disorders (strokes). The severity of vascular dementia depends on how severely the vascular supply is compromised and the location of resulting injuries in the brain.	• Impaired judgment • Impaired ability to make decisions, plan, or organize • May be accompanied by impaired motor function (slow gait and impaired balance)

continues

159

TABLE 6.2 DESCRIPTIONS AND CHARACTERISTICS OF SELECT NEUROCOGNITIVE DISORDERS (CONT.)

GENERAL DESCRIPTION	COMMON FEATURES OR CHARACTERISTICS
CHRONIC TRAUMATIC ENCEPHALOPATHY (CTE)	
Occurs with traumatic brain injury (TBI), including repeated episodes of "mild" TBI with concussions. In late stages, CTE causes profound atrophy of the frontal and medial temporal lobes of the brain and atrophy of the brain's white matter. Characterized by behavioral/psychiatric, cognitive, and motor impairment. CTE has been reported in veterans who have experienced combat and in people who have been involved in contact sports such as football (Fesharaki-Zadeh, 2019).	• **Behavioral and psychiatric domain effects:** Aggression, depression, apathy, impulsivity, delusions including paranoia, and suicidality • **Cognitive domain effects:** Diminished attention and concentration, memory deficits, executive functioning deficits, visuospatial dysfunction, language deficits, and dementia • **Motor domain effects:** Dysarthria, gait abnormalities, ataxia and incoordination, spasticity, and Parkinson's-like symptoms such as tremors
LEWY BODY DISEASE/DEMENTIA WITH LEWY BODIES (DLB)	
Caused by abnormal aggregations or clumps of alpha-synuclein protein neurons in the cerebral cortex. Most patients with DLB also have pathology indicative of AD; about 5 to 10% of people with dementia have DLB alone.	• Symptoms similar to those of AD • Sleep disturbances • Visual hallucinations • Parkinson's-like symptoms such as slowness and gait imbalances

PARKINSON'S DISEASE DEMENTIA (PDD)	
A progressive neurodegenerative disease that affects cognitive status. PDD occurs in individuals with a diagnosis of Parkinson's disease. Estimates of the percentage of people with Parkinson's disease who develop PDD vary widely. The onset of PDD has been reported to be about 10 years after the onset of PD.	• Symptoms similar to those of AD • Impairment in two or more cognitive domains (attention, executive function, memory, or visual function and processing) • Cognitive impairment severe enough to affect daily life (social, occupational, or personal self-care), independent of impairment of motor symptoms of PD • Visual hallucinations • Rapid eye movement sleep behavior disorders • Depression and anxiety

CARING FOR PEOPLE WITH PSYCHIATRIC/ MENTAL HEALTH DISABILITY AND NEUROCOGNITIVE DISORDERS

Nurses who interact with people with PMH disability and neurocognitive disorders must be aware of stereotypes about these populations and of their own biases about them. Nurses must also take steps to provide care based on facts rather than misconceptions.

Healthcare professionals with a background in and experience caring for people with PMH disability are usually well prepared to provide appropriate care for this population. However, *all* healthcare professionals require the knowledge and skills necessary to interact effectively with people with these disorders. People with PMH disability may come in contact with the healthcare system for health issues unrelated to their disability. They need healthcare providers who interact with them without bias and stereotyping and who have the ability to plan and implement appropriate care and treatment.

People with severe PMH disability or neurocognitive disorders require healthcare that addresses their health issues in the context of their disability, but without focusing on the disability to the exclusion of other issues. In other words, the patient's PMH disability or neurocognitive disorder should not be the healthcare provider's only focus, but the nature and severity of the disability or disorder should influence what care is provided and how.

As with all patients in their care, healthcare providers must be alert to possible interactions of medications that patients take to treat PMH issues or neurocognitive disorders with other medications that may be prescribed for the problem for which they are seeking care. It is also important that medication regimens used by patients to treat PMH issues and neurocognitive disorders continue uninterrupted during treatment or hospitalization.

In acute settings, nurses must ensure that admitted patients with PMH disability or a neurocognitive disorder do not pose a risk to themselves or to others to safeguard everyone's safety. In collaboration with other healthcare providers, the nurse's role is to provide emotional support to the patient, orient the patient to the environment, provide prescribed pharmacologic treatments, and provide physical and emotional care and support as indicated.

To ensure the safety of patients with PMH disability or neurocognitive disorders, healthcare providers must also respond to verbal and nonverbal behavioral clues that may indicate that a patient is contemplating self-harm or suicide. Patients with major depression or schizophrenia are at high risk for suicide. The risk of suicide is also increased in patients with a new diagnosis of dementia (Seyfried et al., 2011) as well as patients who feel a sense of hopelessness, anger, frustration, or rejection. Healthcare providers must ask patients who indicate that they have thoughts of suicide or have had them in the past if they have a plan for suicide. Establishing a therapeutic relationship with the patient and asking the patient directly about thoughts of suicide are essential aspects of patient assessment. Providers must also assess whether the patient has the means to commit suicide (e.g., access to firearms, large stashes of medications, knives, or razors). Assessment and close monitoring are of particular importance in older men with neurocognitive disorders who have symptoms of depression or anxiety.

Patients with PMH disability or neurocognitive disorders who are suicidal may require pharmacologic interventions. In addition, these patients need to be cared for by nurses and other healthcare professionals who are warm, sensitive, and consistent in their interactions with the patient. Other strategies to minimize the risk of suicide include the following (Grund, 2018):

- Psychosocial interventions

- Counseling

- Removing items such as glass, cords, shoelaces, razors, toxic/lethal liquids, matches, knives, or nail files that could be used for self-harm

Nurses who feel unable to respond appropriately to patients who are suicidal must obtain immediate consultation with psychiatric nurses or other healthcare providers who are able to respond appropriately to the situation.

After the patient's safety is ensured, it is important to consider the implications of the patient's PMH disability or neurocognitive disorder on the care that is or should be provided to promote the patient's maximum health and well-being. As mentioned, people with PMH disability and neurocognitive disorders often receive inadequate preventive healthcare (e.g., immunizations, cancer screening, smoking-cessation assistance, etc.), general healthcare, and promotion of healthier behaviors and safer environments. Because people with PMH disability and neurocognitive disorders face a high mortality rate and shortened life expectancy, it is essential that healthcare professionals address the prevention and management of chronic medical conditions and the promotion of healthy behaviors with this population.

Nurses and other healthcare providers should not assume that people with PMH disability and neurocognitive disorders are unable or unwilling to participate in health promotion efforts, including preventive health screening. Providing patients with options demonstrates respect for their autonomy and dignity; however, too many options may result in confusion and frustration on the part of the patient. It is also important to consider the cultural norms of a patient with PMH disability or a neurocognitive disorder.

COMMUNICATION STRATEGIES FOR INTERACTING WITH PEOPLE WITH PSYCHIATRIC/MENTAL HEALTH DISABILITY OR NEUROCOGNITIVE DISORDERS

It is important to assess communication strategies used by patients with PMH disability or neurocognitive disorders and to employ appropriate communication strategies when interacting with them (Harwood, 2015). A list of tips follows. (See Chapter 3 for a general overview of strategies for communicating with people with disability.)

- Do not assume a patient is unable to communicate without first conducting an assessment. Every patient's abilities and impairments differ.
- If necessary, obtain information about the patient's communication strategies and style from family members.
- Determine whether a patient has hearing or vision impairment, and ensure assistive devices are available to the patient if needed.
- Speak directly to the patient rather than to an accompanying person.
- Speak clearly and at a normal pace, without overenunciating or shouting.
- Face the patient at eye level and maintain eye contact throughout the conversation. Sit down to communicate with someone seated in a chair or wheelchair.
- Have conversations in quiet, nonstimulating, nondistracting environments.
- Pay attention to the patient's nonverbal communication and behavior.
- Allow time for the patient to understand the question asked.
- Provide ample time for the patient to respond without interruption; don't finish sentences for the patient.
- Encourage patients to share their thoughts.

- Avoid giving false reassurance or minimizing the patient's feelings.
- Avoid giving advice or using language that conveys approval or disapproval.
- Ask one question at a time.
- Allow only one person to speak or ask questions at a time.
- Repeat what the patient said to confirm that you have understood.
- Use concrete language and avoid metaphors, vague terms, and colloquialisms.
- State the patient's (preferred) name to gain the patient's attention.
- If patients become distracted during a conversation, remind them of what they just said or what you were saying or asking.
- Ask questions that require a yes or no response ("Would you like some juice?") rather than questions that require more complex thinking ("What would you like to eat or drink?")
- If verbal communication is impaired, ask the patient to point to what is needed, and use gestures as needed for the purposes of explanation or demonstration.
- Avoid using a patronizing tone of voice or "baby talk"; it is disrespectful, offensive, and usually ineffective.
- Avoid using wording that highlights issues or impairments related to the patient's PMH disability or neurocognitive disorder—for example, "You just asked that question," "I've already answered that question," "Your [spouse, child, other] died many years ago," and so on.
- Do not argue with the patient.
- Avoid using the intercom to communicate.

EDUCATING NURSES TO CARE FOR PEOPLE WITH PSYCHIATRIC/MENTAL HEALTH DISABILITY AND NEUROCOGNITIVE DISORDERS

A number of strategies and resources are available for nurses and other healthcare professionals to increase their knowledge about PMH disability and neurocognitive disorders. Strategies to educate nurses and nursing students about PMH disability and neurocognitive disorders include the following:

- Add content, modules, or courses on PMH disability and neurocognitive disorders to existing curriculum components in classroom, simulation, home care, and clinical experiences.

- Assign students to view and write a report on one of the healthcare stories about people with psychiatric/mental health disability produced by the National Alliance on Mental Illness (https://www.nami.org/videos) and by the UCLA Alzheimer's and Dementia Care Program (https://www.uclahealth.org/dementia/caregiver-education-videos).

- Establish collaborative relationships with agencies and healthcare settings that provide care and services to people with PMH disability and neurocognitive disorders (e.g., community-based mental health services, adult day care centers).

- Initiate clinical sites for and with people with PMH disability and neurocognitive disorders and their families for student clinical assignments and visits. (Provide education to students before first assignment to sites.)

- Identify community agencies with populations of people with PMH disability or neurocognitive disorders to demonstrate for students the ability of people with such conditions to participate in activities, work, and school.

- Invite people with PMH disability or neurocognitive disorders to participate in lectures and panel discussions to enable students to become comfortable asking about these conditions and to learn firsthand about the health-related experiences of people who have them.

- Consider the use of standardized patients in simulations designed to teach learners about communication skills and assessments needed for interacting with individuals with PMH disability or neurocognitive disorders.

If trained actors are used as standardized patients with PMH disability or neurocognitive disorders, ensure that their interactions and behaviors are authentic and avoid stereotyping.

- Build on existing classroom, simulation, home care, and clinical experiences by adding case studies of people with PMH disability and neurocognitive disorders.

- Model positive attitudes, behaviors, and skills toward people with PMH disability and neurocognitive disorders for students.

- Use available resources to better teach students about PMH disability and neurocognitive disorders (see the following sidebar).

- Assign students to identify modifications to patient teaching plans and strategies to accommodate people with varying types and severity of PMH disability and neurocognitive disorders.

- Explore other campus resources, personnel, and faculty who have expertise/experience with people with PMH disability and neurocognitive disorders.

- Participate in disability studies lectures, programs, or courses (if available) on the university or college campus.

- Identify and collaborate with others on campus with a focus on people with disability (e.g., Disabilities Services or Student Services) to identify shared interests and provide mutual support.

- Become active in disability-related organizations in your city or state or on campus to increase visibility and recognition of the need to ensure that all people, including those with PMH disability and neurocognitive disorders, receive appropriate education, healthcare, and services.

- Establish a relationship with people with a PMH disability or neurocognitive disorder in their own environment as well as in a healthcare setting to learn about their everyday issues, challenges, and accomplishments.

- Explore your own creative and innovative approaches to addressing PMH disability and neurocognitive disorders in curriculum. Focus on the day-to-day lives of those affected rather than limiting your focus to acute care issues in hospital settings.

RESOURCES TO TEACH HEALTHCARE PROVIDERS ABOUT PMH DISABILITY AND NEUROCOGNITIVE DISORDERS

- **Arizona Center on Aging: Communicating with Patients Who Have Dementia (https://nursingandhealth.asu.edu/sites/default/files/dementia-patients-communication.pdf):** This is a succinct resource for interprofessional providers on communicating with patients who have dementia.

- **Belfast Health and Social Care Trust: Communicating Effectively with a Person Living with Dementia (http://www.belfasttrust.hscni.net/pdf/dementia_booklet_(2).pdf):** This resource provides detailed suggestions on communicating with people with dementia.

- **Family Caregiver Alliance National Center on Caregiving: Caregiver's Guide to Understanding Dementia Behaviors (https://www.caregiver.org/caregivers-guide-understanding-dementia-behaviors):** This resource provides detailed suggestions on communicating with people with neurocognitive disorders and handling troubling behavior.

- **National Alliance on Mental Illness: Schizophrenia (https://www.nami.org/learn-more/mental-health-conditions/schizophrenia):** This short video illustrates how people with schizophrenia see the world.

- **UCLA Health: Caregiver Training Videos (Alzheimer's and Dementia Care) (https://www.uclahealth.org/dementia/caregiver-education-videos):** This page offers access to informative training videos for caregivers as well as for healthcare providers.

SUMMARY

This chapter discussed issues related to psychiatric/mental health (PMH) disability and neurocognitive disorders. Healthcare professionals often feel uncomfortable interacting with and caring for individuals with these types of disability. Because individuals with PMH disability and neurocognitive disorders can develop general health issues—and indeed are at increased risk for many of them—it is important for all healthcare professionals to be prepared to effectively communicate with these individuals and to provide quality healthcare.

Although PMH disability and neurocognitive disorders are distinct and separate types of disability, some characteristics are similar. Examples of both types of disability were presented and discussed, along with strategies and resources that can be useful in teaching others to provide quality healthcare to people with PMH and neurocognitive disability.

Healthcare providers need to be aware of the stigma associated with PMH disability and neurocognitive disorders and to ensure that care provided does not reflect or reinforce this stigma. They must also ensure that they do not engage in other negative practices that are often experienced by individuals with these disabilities and disorders and their family members.

REFERENCES

ADA Amendments Act of 2008, P.L. 110–325 (2008).

Alzheimer's Association. (2018). 2018 Alzheimer's disease facts and figures. *Alzheimer's & Dementia, 14*(3), 367–429.

American Psychiatric Association. (2015). Diagnostic and statistical manual of mental disorders (DSM-5). Washington, D.C.: Author.

Americans with Disabilities Act of 1990, 42 U.S.C. § 12101 (1990).

Brådvik, L. (2018). Suicide risk and mental disorders. *International Journal of Environmental Research and Public Health, 15*(9), E2028. doi:10.3390/ijerph15092028

Centers for Disease Control and Prevention. (2012). Mental health and chronic diseases. Retrieved from https://www.cdc.gov/workplacehealthpromotion/tools-resources/pdfs/issue-brief-no-2-mental-health-and-chronic-disease.pdf

Centers for Disease Control and Prevention. (2015). Addressing stigma associated with Alzheimer's disease and other dementias: Role of the public health and aging services networks. Retrieved from https://www.cdc.gov/aging/pdf/stigma-and-AD-brief-july-2015.pdf

Conejero, I., Navucet, S., Keller, J., Olié, E., Courtet, P., & Gabelle, A. (2018). A complex relationship between suicide, dementia, and amyloid: A narrative review. *Frontiers in Neuroscience, 12,* 371. doi:10.3389/fnins.2018.00371

Equal Employment Opportunity Commission. (2002). Enforcement guidance: Reasonable accommodation and undue hardship under the Americans with Disabilities Act. Retrieved from https://www.eeoc.gov/policy/docs/accommodation.html

Fesharaki-Zadeh, A. (2019). Chronic traumatic encephalopathy: A brief overview. *Frontiers in Neurology, 10,* 713. doi:10.3389/fneur.2019.00713

Grund, F. J. (2018). Suicide and nonsuicidal self-injury. In M. J. Halter (Ed.), *Varcarolis' foundations of psychiatric mental health nursing: A clinical approach* (pp. 474–489). St. Louis, MO: Elsevier.

Harwood, J. (2015). Communicating with patients who have dementia. Elder Care. Retrieved from https://www.ceadlongisland.org/sites/default/files/Dementia-Patients-Communication.pdf

McCance-Katz, E. F. (2019). The national survey on drug use and health: 2018. Substance Abuse and Mental Health Services Administration (SAMSHA). Retrieved from https://www.samhsa.gov/data/sites/default/files/cbhsq-reports/Assistant-Secretary-nsduh2018_presentation.pdf

National Association of Mental Illness. (2018). The ripple effect of mental illness. Retrieved from https://www.nami.org/NAMI/media/NAMI-Media/Infographics/NAMI-Impact-Ripple-Effect-FINAL.pdf

National Institute of Mental Health. (2018). Statistics. Retrieved from https://www.nimh.nih.gov/health/statistics/index.shtml

National Institute of Mental Health. (2019). Mental illness. Retrieved from https://www.nimh.nih.gov/health/statistics/mental-illness.shtml

National Institute on Aging. (2019). Alzheimer's disease fact sheet. Retrieved from https://www.nia.nih.gov/health/alzheimers-disease-fact-sheet

National Institutes of Health. (2007). NIH curriculum supplement series. Retrieved from https://www.ncbi.nlm.nih.gov/books/NBK20364/

National Rehabilitation Information Center. (2014). What are psychiatric disabilities? Retrieved from https://www.naric.com/?q=en/FAQ/what-are-psychiatric-disabilities

Owens, P. L., Fingar, K. R., McDermott, K. W., Muhri, P. K., & Heslin, K. C. (2019). Inpatient stays involving mental and substance use disorders, 2016. HCUP Statistical Brief #249. Retrieved from www.hcup-us.ahrq.gov/reports/statbriefs/sb249-Mental-Substance-Use-Disorder-Hospital-Stays-2016.pdf

Plassman, B. L., Langa, K. M., Fisher, G. G., Heeringa, S. G., Weir, D. R., Ofstedal, M. B., ... Wallace, R. B. (2007). Prevalence of dementia in the United States: The aging, demographics, and memory study. *Neuroepidemiology, 29*(1–2), 125–132. doi: 10.1159/000109998

Roehrig, C. (2016). Mental disorders top the list of the most costly conditions in the United States: $201 billion. *Health Affairs, 35*(6), 1,130–1,135. doi:10.1377/hlthaff.2015.1659

Ross, C. A., & Goldner, E. M. (2009). Stigma, negative attitudes and discrimination towards mental illness within the nursing profession: A review of the literature. *Journal of Psychiatric and Mental Health Nursing, 16*(6), 558–567. doi:10.1111/j.1365-2850.2009.01399.x

Rudnick, A. (2014). What is a psychiatric disability? *Health Care Analysis, 22*(2), 105–113. doi:10.1007/s10728-012-0235-y

Sachdev, P. S., Blacker, D., Blazer, D. G., Ganguli, M., Jeste, D. V., Paulsen, J. S., & Petersen, R. C. (2014). Classifying neurocognitive disorders: The DSM-5 approach. *Nature Reviews Neurology, 10*(11), 634–642. doi:10.1038/nrneurol.2014.181

Seyfried, L. S., Kales, H. C., Ignacio, R. V., Conwell, Y., & Valenstein, M. (2011). Predictors of suicide in patients with dementia. *Alzheimer's & Dementia, 7*(6), 567–573. doi: 10.1016/j.jalz.2011.01.006

Walker, E. R., McGee, R. E., & Druss, B. G. (2015). Mortality in mental disorders and global disease burden implications: A systematic review and meta-analysis. *JAMA Psychiatry, 72*(4), 334–341. doi:10.1001/jamapsychiatry.2014.2502

World Health Organization. (2015). The epidemiology and impact of dementia: Current state and future trends. Retrieved from https://www.who.int/mental_health/neurology/dementia/dementia_thematicbrief_epidemiology.pdf

World Health Organization. (2017a). Dementia. Retrieved from http://www.who.int/mediacentre/factsheets/fs362/en/

World Health Organization. (2017b). Global action plan on the public health response to dementia 2017–2025. Retrieved from https://apps.who.int/iris/bitstream/handle/10665/259615/9789241513487-eng.pdf;jsessionid=A1026472382AEA6FA8C5295 3469AE089?sequence=1

World Health Organization. (2018a). ICD-11. Retrieved from https://icd.who.int/browse11/l-m/en

World Health Organization. (2018b). Management of physical health conditions in adults with severe mental disorders: WHO guidelines. Retrieved from https://apps.who.int/iris/bitstream/handle/10665/275718/9789241550383-eng.pdf

World Health Organization. (2019). Mental disorders. Retrieved from https://www.who.int/news-room/fact-sheets/detail/mental-disorders

Zembrzuski, C. (2019). Communication difficulties: Assessment and interventions in hospitalized older adults with dementia. Alzheimer's Association. Retrieved from https://consultgeri.org/try-this/dementia/issue-d7.pdf

Zimmerman, M., Morgan, T. A., & Stanton, K. (2018). The severity of psychiatric disorders. *World Psychiatry, 17*(3), 258–275. doi:10.1002/wps.20569

7

SENSORY DISABILITY: HEARING LOSS

INTRODUCTION

An estimated 61 million adults in the US, or one in every 4 adults and 1 in 6 children ages 3 to 17, live with a disability (Centers for Disease Control and Prevention [CDC], 2019; Zablotsky et al., 2019). Among these are disabilities that affect sensory function. Sensory disability affects one or more of the senses (hearing, vision, smell, taste, and *somatosensory*—sensitivity to touch, heat, cold, and painful stimuli) and balance.

People receive 95% of information about the environment around us through our ability to hear and see. So, hearing loss and vision loss affect how we obtain information about the world (National Rehabilitation Information Center, 2019). The focus of this chapter is hearing loss.

Definitions of hearing loss vary somewhat from one source to another. The World Health Organization (WHO, 2019) defines *hearing loss* as an inability to hear as well as someone with normal hearing—that is, someone who has a hearing threshold of 25 decibels (dB) or better in both ears. According to WHO, disabling hearing loss is hearing loss of greater than 40 dB in the better-hearing ear in adults and greater than 30 dB in the better-hearing ear in children. The term *hard of hearing* or *hearing impaired* describes hearing loss that is moderate to severe. People who are hard of hearing or hearing impaired cannot hear sounds under 40 dB in their better ear without the use of a hearing aid or other assistive device. Finally, the term *deaf* describes people with very little or no hearing. This is referred to as profound hearing loss (WHO, 2019).

Others define hearing loss more broadly as the loss of ability to hear sounds.

CHANGES IN TERMINOLOGY OVER TIME

Terminology used to describe people with hearing loss has changed over time. Many people with hearing loss no longer consider the terms *hearing impairment* and *hearing impaired* acceptable. The terms *deaf, hard of hearing,* and *hearing loss* are generally considered more respectful and are preferred by many people with loss of hearing (National Association of the Deaf [NAD], 2020). Many consider *people with hearing loss* to be the most inclusive term, and it is used in this chapter where possible.

It is important to ask people how they prefer to identify themselves. Their preferences may reflect their identification with others with comparable hearing loss. For example, many people who have hearing loss from birth do not see themselves as having lost their hearing; rather, they consider themselves Deaf (with a capital D) and identify with the Deaf community. In turn, some people who became deaf later in life identify themselves as late-deafened with a small d. On a related note, be aware that not all organizations use updated terminology.

The terms *deaf and dumb* and *deaf-mute* are universally offensive. These archaic terms have no place in today's vocabulary. They reflect the unfounded belief that if people are unable to communicate using their voice in the same way that people who are not hard of hearing or deaf do, they are incapable of thinking or learning (NAD, 2020).

The frequency of the sound wave vibration and the sound pressure level dictate the sound pitch and sound level, respectively (The Voice Foundation, n.d.; WHO, 2015). The higher the sound pressure level, the louder the sound. Sound pressure level is measured in decibels (dB). For a sound to be heard by the human ear, it must be above a certain decibel level, or threshold (Institute for Quality and Efficiency in Health Care [IQWiG], 2017). Following are examples of the volume, or loudness, of familiar sounds, in decibels:

- Quiet countryside: 2 dB
- Quiet conversation: 40 dB
- Normal conversation: 60 dB
- Traffic: 80 dB

- Industrial noise: 100 dB
- Very loud music: 120 dB
- Nearby thunder: 120 dB
- Jet engine: 140 dB

Daily or continuous exposure to sounds above 90 dB—such as industrial noise (say, from a jackhammer), very loud music, and jet engine sounds—can lead to hearing loss. Sounds louder than 110 dB are uncomfortable; those over 130 dB produce pain and can cause acute hearing loss (IQWiG, 2017).

As noted, a person who can hear, but not as well as someone with normal hearing, is said to have hearing loss. Loss of hearing of 20 dB or more below the hearing threshold constitutes some degree of hearing loss. The degree or extent of hearing loss may be mild, moderate, moderate-severe, severe, or profound. It can affect one ear (*unilateral*) or both ears (*bilateral*), and there may be differences in the degree of hearing loss between the ears. Categories or degrees of hearing and hearing loss have been reported as follows (2017):

- Normal hearing: Hearing loss of 0 to 25 dB
- Mild hearing loss: Hearing loss of 26 to 40 dB
- Moderate hearing loss: Hearing loss of 41 to 55 dB
- Moderate-severe hearing loss: Hearing loss of 56 to 70 dB
- Severe hearing loss: Hearing loss of 71 to 90 dB
- Profound hearing loss or deafness: Hearing loss of more than 90 dB

With moderate to severe hearing loss, people are unable to hear and repeat words spoken in a normal voice (WHO, 2019).

People who are hard of hearing usually communicate through spoken language. They may benefit from hearing aids, cochlear implants, and other assistive devices, as well as captioning. Those with more severe hearing loss and those who are Deaf often use sign language for communication, although some may benefit from cochlear implants. These assistive devices are discussed later in this chapter.

> Hearing loss has a great impact on a child's development and on the ability of adults to interact with others and their environment.

PREVALENCE OF HEARING LOSS

WHO (2019) defines *disabling hearing loss* as hearing loss greater than 40 dB in the better-hearing ear in adults and greater than 30 dB in the better-hearing ear in children. According to WHO (2019), more than 466 million people, or 5% of the world's population, have disabling hearing loss. Disabling hearing loss affects 432 million adults and 34 million children. WHO (2019) estimates that by 2050, more than 900 million to 1 billion people, or 1 in every 10 people, will have disabling hearing loss. Further, one-third of people over the age of 65 have disabling hearing loss.

According to the National Institute on Deafness and Other Communication Disorders (NIDCD, 2016), hearing loss is common, and it is increasing over time. It has been identified as the fifth leading cause of years lived with a disability on a global level (National Academies of Sciences, Engineering, and Medicine [NASEM], 2016).

Specific statistics from NIDCD (2016) related to hearing loss in the US in adults are as follows:

- Approximately 15% of American adults (37.5 million) age 18 and over report some hearing loss.

- Approximately 13% of people in the US (30 million) age 12 years or older have hearing loss in both ears, based on standard hearing examinations.

- Disabling hearing loss occurs in 2% of adults age 45 to 54, 8.5% of adults age 55 to 64, 25% of adults age 65 to 74, and 50% of adults age 75 and older.

- Age is the strongest predictor of hearing loss among adults age 20 to 69, with the greatest amount of hearing loss in the 60–69 age group.

- Hearing loss occurs twice as often in men than women age 20 to 69.

- Non-Hispanic white adults are more likely than other racial/ethnic groups to have hearing loss.

- Non-Hispanic Black adults have the lowest prevalence of hearing loss among adults age 20 to 69.

NIDCD (2016) statistics on hearing loss in the US among children are as follows:

- Between 2 and 3 of every 1,000 children in the United States have a detectable level of hearing loss at birth in one or both ears.

- More than 90% of Deaf children are born to hearing parents.

- 60% of hearing loss in children is due to preventable causes.

In addition, according to the NIDCD (2016), three of every five children younger than 5 years of age globally are at risk for not reaching their developmental potential because of hearing loss. In a recent international study of developmental disability among children, hearing loss was the most prevalent disability after vision loss, intellectual disability, and autism spectrum disorder (Global Research on Developmental Disabilities Collaborators, 2018).

The prevalence of sensory losses like hearing loss is expected to increase in the US as its population ages. As a result, minimizing the impact of sensory disability takes on increasing importance to maintain independent living, health, and quality of life among adults as they age (Dillon, Gu, Hoffman, & Ko, 2010). Because of the prevalence of hearing loss and the likelihood that nurses in all clinical settings will encounter patients with hearing loss, it is important to address these issues within the discussion of disability.

CAUSES OF HEARING LOSS

To understand hearing loss, one must understand how hearing works:

1. The movement of objects—e.g., the vibration of strings on a musical instrument, the vibration of a person's vocal cord when speaking or singing, cars passing by, etc.—generates sound waves.

2. The outer ear *(pinna)* and middle ear amplify sound waves.

3. The amplified sound waves cause the ear drum (tympanic membrane) to vibrate.

4. Sensory cells in the cochlea, located in the inner ear, convert these vibrations to electrical nerve signals.

5. The electrical nerve signals are transmitted to the brain.

6. The brain analyzes the nerve signals, recognizes them as sounds, and interprets them as music, speaking or singing, or traffic noise.

Hearing loss occurs when cochlea sensory cells are damaged. There is a fixed number of these cells present at birth. When these cells are damaged, they do not regenerate, resulting in hearing loss.

Hearing loss, which may occur at any age, can be sudden or gradual, can affect one or both ears, and can affect one or more components of the auditory system that are involved in hearing. Causes of hearing loss are categorized as acquired or congenital.

Causes of *acquired hearing loss* include the following:

* Aging (a major cause of acquired hearing loss)

* Trauma

* Excessive noise exposure (e.g., occupational or recreational noise; lack of ear protection; personal audio devices at high volumes and for prolonged periods of time; and regular attendance at concerts, nightclubs, bars, and sporting events, causing damage to the cilia of the inner ear)

* Infectious disease (e.g., meningitis, measles, or mumps)

* Exposure to ototoxic medications

* Chronic ear infections (a common cause of hearing loss among children)

* Cerumen (wax) or foreign bodies blocking the ear canal

Causes of *congenital hearing loss* include the following:

* Birth complications

* Infectious disease affecting pregnant women (e.g., maternal rubella, syphilis, and others)

* Low birth weight

* Birth asphyxia

* Maternal use of ototoxic medications (e.g., aminoglycosides, cytotoxic drugs, antimalarial drugs, and diuretics)

* Various neurodegenerative disorders and syndromes

* Hereditary and nonhereditary genetic factors

Although adults with age-related hearing loss (referred to as *presbycusis*) can benefit from treatment, hearing loss in adults is usually permanent and often goes untreated. At least 75% of people

More than 400 genes that cause hearing loss have been identified to date (McKee, Schlehofer, & Thew, 2013).

with hearing loss do not receive treatment that could be beneficial in communication and in overcoming barriers associated with hearing loss (McKee, Lin, & Zazove, 2018).

More than 60% of cases of hearing loss can be attributed to preventable causes. Preventable hearing loss occurs in 75% of children under 15 years of age in low- and middle-income countries and 49% in high-income countries. Because of its pervasiveness, prevention of excessive noise exposure has become a major goal of the World Health Organization (NIDCD, 2018; WHO, 2015, 2019).

CONSEQUENCES OF HEARING LOSS

Major consequences of hearing loss include effects on communication, social interactions, and participation in one's community. Hearing loss among older adults—an expanding population—is associated with cognitive decline and neurocognitive disorders, falls, decreased physical functioning, and hospitalization. In both children and adults, the effects of hearing loss on social and emotional well-being can be significant and can result in feelings of loneliness, isolation, and frustration (WHO, 2019).

Financial costs associated with hearing loss include reduced income, unemployment and underemployment, and costs related to treatment of hearing loss (NASEM, 2016; WHO, 2019). Costs also include those associated with educational support—for example, teaching people sign language—and providing educational assistance and certified sign language interpreters when needed. WHO (2015) reports that global costs associated with healthcare services to address hearing loss and related lost productivity amount to $750–790 billion

Hearing loss is often an invisible disability. That is, it is not always obvious to others. So, there is a risk that a person's hearing loss may go unrecognized for years, with the person receiving no treatment or services to address functional, social, and educational needs.

annually. These costs are expected to rise due to a global population that is both growing (an estimated 9 billion people by 2050) and aging.

Hearing sounds and words helps children learn to talk and to understand others. Acquisition of speech and language begins in the first few months of life. So, early hearing loss affects communication and social skills. Children with profound hearing loss before acquiring spoken language—which generally occurs by age 2—often have difficultly speaking clearly. Severe hearing loss in young children may result in delayed speech and language skills; difficulty reading, learning in school, and interacting with other children; and poor self-esteem. In addition, because of the role of hearing and speech in achieving developmental milestones, undetected or delayed diagnosis and treatment of hearing loss in children often results in other developmental delays.

Hearing loss can affect the academic performance of children if they do not receive educational assistance and accommodations. Assistive devices, discussed later in this chapter, can enhance the development of speech and language in children if used very early in life.

The inability of some people with hearing loss to adequately communicate health issues to healthcare providers often results in these issues going untreated, further affecting their functional and health status. This is made worse by a lack of understanding among healthcare professionals of the significant impact of hearing loss and their failure to accommodate the communication, teaching, and healthcare needs of people who are deaf or hard of hearing.

Another important consequence of hearing loss is low health literacy. *Health literacy* refers to people's ability to obtain, process, understand, and use basic health information and services to make appropriate health-related decisions. WHO identifies health literacy as central to health and states that inclusive and equitable access to education and lifelong learning is foundational to health literacy (WHO, 2017). People with acquired hearing loss due to aging or with profound hearing loss from an early age are at high risk for low levels of health literacy. Communication barriers associated with hearing loss, lack of education, and limited access to health-related information tailored to the Deaf or those with hearing loss make this an important issue. In particular, people in the Deaf community may not have basic knowledge about health issues because of their lack of access to public service announcements and health-related messages in a language they can understand. American Sign Language (ASL) users experience many communication barriers that limit their access to information, which results in low awareness and understanding of common health issues, as well as health-promotion strategies to minimize the impact of these health issues, on their well-being and health (McKee et al., 2013; McKee et al., 2015; Richardson, 2014; WHO, 2017). This has major implications for clinicians, who often expect patients to have a certain level of knowledge about health-related issues and health risks.

Although hearing loss does not cause balance disorders, some people with hearing loss also experience vertigo and other balance problems because the inner ear is responsible for both hearing and vestibular (proprioception and balance) function.

CHARACTERISTICS OF HEARING LOSS

There are several ways to categorize hearing loss. As discussed previously, one way to categorize hearing loss is by whether it is acquired or congenital. Another is by severity: mild, moderate, moderate-severe, severe, or profound (WHO, 2019).

Hearing loss can also be categorized by age of onset—or, more precisely, level of speech and language skills at onset. Hearing loss that occurs before a child acquires speech and language skills (generally around age 2) is called *prelingual hearing loss* or *deafness*. This type of hearing loss or deafness usually prevents the person from speaking clearly unless they receive cochlear implants and speech therapy very early in life. Hearing loss that occurs after a person acquires speech and language skills is called *post-lingual hearing loss* or *deafness*. People with post-lingual hearing loss or deafness are usually able to speak clearly.

Finally, hearing loss can be categorized by the part of the hearing apparatus that is affected. These categories are conductive, sensorineural, and mixed. Table 7.1 describes each of these categories in more detail.

TABLE 7.1 CONDUCTIVE, SENSORINEURAL, AND MIXED HEARING LOSS

CATEGORY OF HEARING LOSS	CLINICAL FEATURES AND TREATMENT
CONDUCTIVE HEARING LOSS	
Caused by factors that prevent sound from passing through the outer or middle ear to the inner ear. These could include fluid in the middle ear due to infection or allergy, otitis media, punctured tympanic membrane, a benign tumor that blocks the external or middle ear, an accumulation of cerumen (wax) in the ear canal, malformation of the external or middle ear structures, or obstruction of the Eustachian tube.	• Conductive hearing loss can occur at any age. • Conductive hearing loss can often be treated with medicine or surgery. • Treatment depends on the cause of the hearing loss.
SENSORINEURAL HEARING LOSS	
Caused by damage to the inner ear (cochlea) or auditory nerve. This could be due to illness (such as autoimmune disease of the inner ear), ototoxic medication, familial hearing loss, aging, exposure to loud noises, head trauma, malformation of the inner ear, Ménière's disease, or otosclerosis (abnormal remodeling of the small bones of the inner ear with impaired vibration and transmission of vibrations necessary for hearing).	• Hearing aids may be helpful in some cases. • If hearing aids are inadequate, sensorineural hearing loss can be treated effectively with cochlear implants.

MIXED HEARING LOSS	
A combination of conductive (damage to outer or middle ear) and sensorineural (damage to inner ear or auditory nerve) hearing loss.	• Treatment strategies depend on the severity of each type of hearing loss. • Treatment may be a combination of approaches described above.

CARING FOR PEOPLE WITH DISABILITY DUE TO HEARING LOSS

Like people with other types of disability, those with hearing loss and deafness are at risk for bias, stigma, and stereotyping. In addition to affecting their integration and participation in society, education, and work settings, this results in inequitable healthcare. Lack of knowledge and understanding among healthcare professionals of the perspectives of people who are hard of hearing or Deaf further contributes to low-quality healthcare.

The stigma associated with loss of hearing due to aging is one reason that many people who could benefit from hearing aids are reluctant or refuse to wear them.

Nurses and other healthcare professionals must understand that members of the Deaf community (people with profound hearing loss, usually from birth) do not consider themselves to have a disability. Further, their first and often only language is ASL. ASL has no written form (McKee et al., 2013). Only about 20% of Deaf people are proficient in written English, and the average English reading level among Deaf high school seniors is estimated to be at or below a fourth-grade reading level (McKee et al., 2013). It is also worth noting that those who use lip-reading (watching people's lips as they speak to interpret what they are saying) or speech-reading (doing lip-reading while also watching the speaker's facial expressions and gestures) generally recognize only about 10 to 30% of spoken language (Altieri, Pisoni, & Townsend, 2011). This has serious implications for nurses, who generally provide teaching, health promotion, and discharge instructions for patients (McKee et al., 2015).

If healthcare providers know ahead of time that they will be interacting with or caring for someone with hearing loss, they should address that person's communication needs ahead of time. For example, if the person's primary method of communication is sign language, this might mean providing a certified ASL interpreter. Similarly, if a person who uses lip-reading or speech-reading is scheduled for a procedure such as an MRI or mammogram, during which the healthcare provider's face might not be visible to the patient, or one during which the healthcare provider will be wearing a surgical mask, the procedure should be explained to the patient beforehand. Such patients should be told what they will experience during the procedure, what they will be expected to do, and what support and assistance will be available to them and when (before, during, or after the procedure). This might involve using videos, pictures, and other means of communicating information and instruction. This ensures that people with hearing loss understand the procedure they are about to undergo and have the information they need to make decisions and to follow instructions.

According to Alexander, Ladd, and Powell (2012), 87% of clinicians report confidence in their ability to communicate with members of the Deaf community. However, members of the Deaf community report poor access and communication with healthcare clinicians (Alexander et al., 2012). Therefore, healthcare professionals should not be overly confident in their ability to communicate with members of the Deaf community.

It's important for nurses and other healthcare professionals to be aware that the Americans with Disabilities Act (ADA) requires healthcare facilities to provide effective means of communication for patients, family members, and hospital visitors who are deaf or hard of hearing (US Department of Justice [USDOJ], 2003). This applies to all hospital programs and services, including emergency departments, inpatient and outpatient services and clinics, surgery, educational classes and sessions, cafeterias, and gift shops (USDOJ,

2003). When needed, certified ASL interpreters should be provided. The ADA mandates that the healthcare facility cover costs associated with providing such services.

In its "Position Statement on Healthcare Access for Deaf Patients," the National Association of the Deaf (NAD, n.d.) notes that lack of accessible healthcare and effective communication for this population likely result in the following:

- Longer hospital stays

- More emergency department visits

- More hospital readmissions

- Poor healthcare follow-up

- Low levels of treatment adherence

- Poor health outcomes

- Low levels of patient satisfaction

NAD (n.d.) recommends the following strategies for healthcare clinicians to improve care provided to Deaf patients:

- Clearly identify people at risk for poor communication.

- Use visual medical aids (such as charts, diagrams, and models) to explain concepts and anatomy, as well as online resources to reinforce teaching and understanding.

- Learn basic sign language. (Although years of training are needed for fluency, being able to use at least some sign language may make Deaf patients more comfortable.)

- Establish and follow a policy to ask patients who are hard of hearing or deaf about their communication needs to ensure appropriate care at subsequent visits.

- Use qualified sign language interpreters (not family members).

- Avoid ineffective methods of communication.

- Do not assume that lip-reading, speech-reading, and note-writing are effective.

- Use available patient-education programs and teach-back strategies to ensure that patients understand information and instruction. (Do not assume that if patients nod their heads they understand.)

- Become familiar with and adhere to relevant laws that mandate equal access and communication for all, including those who are deaf and hard of hearing.

The specific strategies needed to ensure effective communication are determined by the needs of the person with hearing loss. Healthcare providers should not assume without asking what people with hearing loss require or prefer. If written notes are acceptable to those with hearing loss, those notes should be destroyed to protect their privacy.

Family members are not appropriate as interpreters because of privacy concerns, because they may be unfamiliar with terminology and unable to interpret accurately, and because they may be unable to interpret in emergency situations.

People who have low health literacy due to hearing loss are at increased risk for health disorders due to their lack of knowledge about health issues, health-promotion strategies, and preventive health screening. It is important for nurses to address health promotion with people who are hard of hearing or deaf. Healthcare professionals should not assume people with hearing loss are uninterested or unable to participate. Although hearing loss may not be the focus of a healthcare visit or hospitalization, it should not be ignored. The effects of hearing loss on a person's ability to obtain healthcare and healthcare information should be addressed as part of nursing care.

Clinicians often expect a certain level of knowledge about health-related issues and health risks. Patients who have hearing loss might not have such knowledge due to low health literacy.

RECOMMENDED STRATEGIES FOR COMMUNICATING WITH PEOPLE WHO ARE DEAF OR HARD OF HEARING

- Identify and honor the communication preferences of the person who is hard of hearing or deaf.
- Face the person directly, at eye level, and in good light.
- Have conversations in a room with as little extraneous noise as possible.
- Talk directly to the person and not the interpreter or other accompanying person.
- Use the person's name to gain the person's attention.
- Speak in a normal tone of voice, without shouting or exaggerating mouth movements.
- Do not speak rapidly or use lengthy or complicated sentences.
- Do not turn away when speaking.
- Keep your hands away from your face while talking.
- Avoid doing other things when talking. This is likely to be distracting to the person and interfere with the ability to pay attention to what you are saying.
- If the listener hears better in one ear than the other, direct the conversation to that ear.
- Rephrase wording as needed to clarify issues rather than repeating the same wording if you are not understood.
- If you are giving specific information—such as a time, place, or phone number—to people who are hard of hearing or deaf, verify that they heard the information correctly.
- Provide important information—such as directions, schedules, medication dosages, and follow-up healthcare visits—in writing or some other alternative format.
- Recognize that someone who is hard of hearing or deaf may have a harder time understanding when ill, stressed, or tired.
- Watch for puzzled looks or other body language or facial expressions that may indicate a misunderstanding. If you see these, tactfully ask if the person understood you or ask leading questions so you know your message got across.

Many people with hearing loss use assistive devices to hear and understand spoken language, although the sound is usually not what might be considered "normal speech." Users of these devices usually need some period of time, and perhaps some amount of rehabilitation or therapy, to become accustomed to them and to understand what they are hearing. Table 7.2 identifies and briefly describes such devices and when they might be used.

TABLE 7.2   ASSISTIVE HEARING DEVICES

DEVICES AND DESCRIPTIONS	INDICATIONS AND COMMENTS
HEARING AIDS	
Electronic devices that amplify sound. Hearing aids are worn in or behind the ear. They receive sound waves through a microphone, convert them to electrical signals, and send them to an amplifier, which increases the power of the signals and sends them to the ear through a receiver or speaker.	Hearing aids amplify sounds and make it possible for people to hear and understand them better. However, only one of every five people who could benefit from a hearing aid actually uses one. Hearing aids can be worn by people of any age, including infants. Infants who have hearing loss and use hearing aids may be better able to hear and understand sounds, which increases their likelihood of developing language and speech at a young age. Young children are usually fitted with behind-the-ear hearing aids to accommodate growth.
BONE-ANCHORED HEARING AIDS	
Devices that require the insertion of a titanium rod into the mastoid portion of the temporal bone. The rod is then connected to a bone conduction hearing aid to enable direct vibration transmission to the skull.	This type of hearing aid may be used when a child has conductive, mixed, or unilateral hearing loss. It may be especially suitable for children who cannot otherwise wear or tolerate the usual type of hearing aid. This type of hearing aid has been used with congenital malformations of the external and middle ear, chronically discharging ears, and conductive hearing loss due to ossicular disease. This type of hearing aid is expensive because of costs of the device and the surgical procedure required.

COCHLEAR IMPLANT DEVICES

Surgically implanted electronic devices that send sound signals directly to the auditory nerve, bypassing components of the ear that may be damaged or missing. These devices have internal and external components. External components include a microphone, battery, speech processor, external magnet, and transmitter antenna. Internal components include an internal magnet, antenna, receiver-stimulator, and electrode array.

These are used in cases of sensorineural deafness. They may allow some people who are deaf to learn to hear and interpret sounds and speech. Cochlear implants do not amplify sounds. The implantation of these devices is generally a low-risk outpatient procedure. Candidates for cochlear implants now include children as young as 1 year old with profound prelingual and postlingual hearing loss and deafness, and those with greater degrees of residual hearing.

Some members of the Deaf community view cochlear implants in a negative light. They see them as an effort to impose the values of others on the Deaf community and to decrease the size of the community. Healthcare professionals often strongly disagree with parents of children with profound hearing loss who reject the use of cochlear implants. However, clinicians must respect their decision and work with them and their child to provide the highest-quality care possible.

AUDITORY BRAINSTEM IMPLANT

A device that bypasses the inner ear and auditory nerve and directly stimulates hearing pathways in the brainstem. These devices have internal and external components.

This device can be used to treat severe to profound hearing loss due to an absent or very small auditory nerve or severely abnormal inner ear (cochlea) when a hearing aid or cochlear implant is not effective. Implanting this device requires a craniotomy, and the outcomes are highly variable. Thus, it is not the first line of treatment.

Clinicians should be aware of any assistive devices used by patients for whom they provide care. They should also ensure that these devices are used when communicating with these patients and are protected from loss or damage when not in use.

Be cautious with patients who have an implanted assistive device in MRI machines. The MRI magnet may damage, displace, or inactivate some of these devices, causing discomfort or pain, although MRIs can be safely used with some newer devices. Ensure that the radiology department is aware of any patients who have an implanted device and that the MRI is safe for these patients.

People with hearing loss and deafness may be adept at using other means to communicate, including electronic and nonelectronic assistive devices. These include the following:

- Group and personal FM amplification systems
- Inductive loop amplification systems ("pocket talker")
- Infrared amplification systems
- Telephone amplifiers
- Nonelectronic approaches

In addition, recent advances in technology have enabled the use of smartphones, computers, and other devices to augment hearing aids (McKee et al., 2018). Other tools include communication boards with pictures and computer programs that synthesize speech from text or pictures. These can be helpful means for people with hearing loss and healthcare professionals to communicate more effectively. Speech-to-text technology and communication access real-time translation (CART) or captioning are other approaches to promote communication and understanding between people with hearing loss and healthcare professionals.

EDUCATING NURSES TO CARE FOR PEOPLE WITH HEARING LOSS

A number of strategies and resources are available for nurses and other healthcare professionals to increase their knowledge about hearing loss. These include the following:

- Add content, modules, or courses on hearing loss and deafness to existing curriculum components in classroom, simulation, home care, and clinical experiences.

- Assign students to view and write a report on one of the healthcare stories about people with hearing loss and deafness, available from https://www.medel.com/about-hearing/hearing-loss-stories.

- Assign students to read a story on the experience of a child with hearing loss at https://www.rchsd.org/health-articles/hearing-impairment-kristins-story/.

- Establish collaborative relationships with agencies or healthcare settings that provide care and services to people with hearing loss and deafness (e.g., schools for the deaf, Deaf Community Services; centers for independent living).

- Initiate clinical sites for and with people with hearing loss and deafness and their families for student clinical assignments and visits. (Provide education to students before first assignment to sites.)

- Identify community agencies with populations of people with hearing loss or deafness to demonstrate for students the ability of people with such conditions to participate in activities, work, and school.

- Invite people with hearing loss or deafness to participate in lectures and panel discussions to enable students to become comfortable asking about these conditions and to learn firsthand about the health-related experiences of people who have them (after ensuring that appropriate communication strategies, including ASL interpreters, are available).

- Explore the inclusion of people with hearing loss or deafness as standardized patients in

Only people with hearing loss or deafness should serve as hearing loss/deafness standardized patients. This ensures authentic experiences and prevents stereotyping.

simulations. Provide training so that expectations are clear to those with hearing loss or deafness, faculty, staff, and students.

- Build on existing classroom, simulation, home care, and clinical experiences by adding case studies of people with hearing loss and deafness.

- Model positive attitudes, behaviors, and skills for students toward people with hearing loss or deafness.

- Use available resources to better teach students about hearing disability (see the following sidebar).

- Assign students to identify modifications to patient teaching plans and strategies to accommodate people with varying types and severity of hearing loss.

- Explore other campus resources, personnel, and faculty who have expertise/experience with people with hearing loss.

- Participate in disability studies lectures, programs, or courses (if available) on the university or college campus.

- Identify and collaborate with others on campus with a focus on people with disability (e.g., Disabilities Services or Student Services) to identify shared interests and provide mutual support.

- Become active in disability-related organizations in your city or state or on campus to increase visibility and recognition of the need to ensure that all people, including those with hearing loss or deafness, receive appropriate education, healthcare, and services.

- Establish a relationship with people with hearing loss or deafness in their own environment as well as in a healthcare setting to learn about their everyday issues, challenges, and accomplishments.

- Explore and develop your own creative and innovative approaches to addressing hearing loss disability in curriculum. Focus on the day-to-day lives of those affected rather than limiting your focus to acute care issues in hospital settings.

RESOURCES TO TEACH HEALTHCARE PROVIDERS ABOUT HEARING LOSS DISABILITY

- **Curbside Consultation: Caring for Older Patients Who Have Significant Hearing Loss (https://www.aafp.org/afp/2013/0301/p360. pdf):** This article provides a brief, focused discussion of primary care for older people with hearing loss.

- **Hearing Loss Association of America (HLAA): Guide for Effective Communication in Health Care for Providers (https://www. hearingloss.org/wp-content/uploads/HLAA_HC_Providers_ Complete_Guide.pdf):** This is a detailed guide for healthcare clinicians who may interact with people with hearing loss in many settings. It includes a communication access plan (CAP), which is a one-page form to inform clinicians about hearing status and communication aids.

- **Hearing Loss Association of America (HLAA): Technology (https:// www.hearingloss.org/hearing-help/technology):** This website provides a detailed discussion and illustrations of assistive technology used by people with hearing loss.

- **National Association for the Deaf (NAD) Position Statements (https://www.nad.org/about-us/position-statements):** This site offers a number of position statements on issues related to hearing loss.

- **National Association for the Deaf Resources (https://www.nad.org/ resources):** This page includes a list of resources for people with hearing loss and healthcare professionals.

- **Hearing Loss Association of America: Technology for Patients (https://www.youtube.com/watch?v=lXbfs9iQhug&feature=you tu.be):** This brief video offers communication strategies and technologies to make hospital trips easier for people with hearing loss.

SUMMARY

People with hearing loss or deafness are often evaluated and treated for these issues in specialty clinics or practices. However, given the sizable population of people with these disabling conditions, healthcare professionals are very likely to interact with people with hearing impairment in other healthcare settings. Healthcare professionals who are knowledgeable about these conditions and familiar with strategies to effectively communicate with people with hearing loss are likely to be able to effectively identify and address their healthcare needs. They are also more likely to be able to use or develop strategies to teach and prepare them for procedures or discharge from a hospital or outpatient setting. Healthcare professionals who provide care for people with hearing loss or deafness must be prepared to address their immediate healthcare needs while also considering how hearing impairment might affect their ability to obtain care and communicate with others. Healthcare professionals should also identify people with hearing loss who have not been diagnosed as such and help guide them to receive effective treatment.

REFERENCES

Alexander, A., Ladd, P., & Powell, S. (2012). Deafness might damage your health. *The Lancet, 379*(9820), 979–981. doi:10.1016/S0140-6736(11)61670-X

Altieri, N. A., Pisoni, D. B., & Townsend, J. T. (2011). Some normative data on lip-reading skills (L). *The Journal of the Acoustical Society of America, 130*(1), 1–4. doi: 10.1121/1.3593376

Centers for Disease Control and Prevention. (2019). Disability impacts all of us. Retrieved from https://www.cdc.gov/ncbddd/disabilityandhealth/infographic-disability-impacts-all.html

Dillon, C. F., Gu, Q., Hoffman, H. J., & Ko, C. (2010). Vision, hearing, balance, and sensory impairment in Americans aged 70 years and over: United States, 1999–2006. NCHS Data Brief No. 31. Retrieved from https://www.cdc.gov/nchs/products/databriefs/db31.htm

Eichwald, J. (2017). Adult hearing loss: Recent data from the CDC. Federal Trade Commission Workshop in Washington, D.C. Retrieved from https://www.ftc.gov/system/files/documents/public_events/1022593/eichwald_1.pdf

Global Research on Developmental Disabilities Collaborators. (2018). Developmental disabilities among children younger than 5 years in 195 countries and territories, 1990–2016: A systematic analysis for the Global Burden of Disease Study 2016. *Lancet Global Health, 6*(10), e1100–1121. doi:10.1016/S2214-109X(18)30309-7

Institute for Quality and Efficiency in Health Care. (2017). *Hearing loss and deafness: Normal hearing and impaired hearing.* Retrieved from https://www.ncbi.nlm.nih.gov/books/NBK390300/?report=printable

McKee, M. M., Lin, F. R., & Zazove, P. (2018). State of research and program development for adults with hearing loss. *Disability and Health Journal, 11*(4), 518–524. doi:10.1016/j.dhjo.2018.07.010

McKee, M. M., Paasche-Orlow, M. K., Winters, P. C., Fiscella, K., Zazove, P., Sen, A., & Pearson, T. (2015). Assessing health literacy in Deaf American Sign Language users. *Journal of Health Communication, 20*(Suppl. 2), 92–100. doi:10.1080/10810730.2015.1066468

McKee, M., Schlehofer, D., & Thew, D. (2013). Ethical issues in conducting research with deaf populations. *American Journal of Public Health, 103*(12), 2,174–2,178. doi:10.2105/AJPH.2013.301343

National Academies of Sciences, Engineering, and Medicine. (2016). *Hearing health care for adults: Priorities for improving access and affordability.* Washington, D.C.: The National Academies Press.

National Association of the Deaf. (n.d.). Position statement on health care access for deaf patients. Retrieved from https://www.nad.org/about-us/position-statements/position-statement-on-health-care-access-for-deaf-patients/

National Association of the Deaf. (2020). Community and culture—Frequently asked questions. Retrieved from https://www.nad.org/resources/american-sign-language/community-and-culture-frequently-asked-questions/

National Institute on Deafness and Other Communication Disorders. (2016). Quick statistics about hearing. Retrieved from https://www.nidcd.nih.gov/health/statistics/quick-statistics-hearing

National Institute on Deafness and Other Communication Disorders. (2018). Age-related hearing loss. Retrieved from https://www.nidcd.nih.gov/health/age-related-hearing-loss

National Rehabilitation Information Center. (2019). What are sensory disabilities? Retrieved from https://naric.com/sites/default/files/Sensory%20Disabilities_0.pdf

Richardson, K. J. (2014). Deaf culture: Competencies and best practices. *The Nurse Practitioner, 39*(5), 20–28. doi:10.1097/01.NPR.0000445956.21045.c4

US Department of Justice. (2003). Communicating with people who are deaf or hard of hearing in hospital settings. ADA Business Brief. Retrieved from https://www.ada.gov/hospcombrprt.pdf

The Voice Foundation. (n.d.). Learning about the voice mechanism. Retrieved from https://voicefoundation.org/health-science/voice-disorders/anatomy-physiology-of-voice-production/the-voice-mechanism/

World Health Organization. (2015). Hearing loss due to recreational exposure to loud sounds: A review. Retrieved from https://apps.who.int/iris/bitstream/handle/10665/154589/9789241508513_eng.pdf;sequence=1

World Health Organization. (2017). The mandate for health literacy. Retrieved from https://www.who.int/healthpromotion/conferences/9gchp/health-literacy/en/

World Health Organization. (2019). Deafness and hearing loss. Retrieved from https://www.who.int/news-room/fact-sheets/detail/deafness-and-hearing-loss

Zablotsky, B., Black, L. I., Maenner, M. J., Schieve, L. A., Danielson, M. L., Bitsko, R. H., ... Boyle, C. A. (2019). Prevalence and trends of developmental disabilities among children in the United States: 2009–2017. *Pediatrics, 144*(4), e20190811. doi: 10.1542/peds.2019-0811

8

SENSORY DISABILITY: VISION LOSS

INTRODUCTION

Like the ability to hear, the ability to see helps determine how people perceive and interpret the world. Vision is important to our ability to communicate as well as to our physical health, independence, mobility, social and community participation, education and employment, socioeconomic status, and performance of activities (National Academies of Sciences, Engineering, and Medicine [NASEM], 2016). Vision has a crucial role in every aspect of life. It is a critical component of personal encounters in which information is often shared through nonverbal cues such as gestures, facial expressions, and body language (World Health Organization [WHO], 2019b). In one survey, more than 70% of respondents identified loss of vision as one of the most feared health outcomes (National Eye Institute [NEI], 2019b).

Vision is essential to child development from a very early age—when infants begin to visually recognize and respond to parents, family members, and others. It plays a role in the cognitive and social development of infants and young children, as well as in the development of motor skills, coordination, and balance (WHO, 2019b). Vision is important in education, friendships with others, self-esteem and well-being, and participation in sports, physical activities, and social activities recognized as essential to physical development and to mental and physical health.

Vision loss and blindness can hamper the performance of everyday activities, including walking, reading, caring for others, and functioning in the world. In a world based around the ability to see, vision impairment can have significant consequences for people, their families, and those who provide healthcare (WHO, 2019b).

Vision plays a role in people's personal identity and socialization. With impaired or no vision, these can be negatively affected.

NASEM (2016) describes *vision loss* as the result of physiological changes or structural, neurological, or acquired damage to the structure or function of one or both eyes or to visual information processing structures in the brain. According to the World Health Organization (WHO, 2019b), disability due to vision loss is an impairment, limitation, or restriction that individuals with vision loss experience in their interaction with the physical, social, or attitudinal environment.

A WORD ON THE TERM VISION LOSS

The term *vision loss* suggests a decrease in visual ability and function. However, some people with congenital or very early blindness do not perceive vision impairment as a loss. This view could affect their willingness to accept treatment to improve or even reverse impairment. Still, this chapter uses the term *vision loss*, along with *vision impairment*. Neither term is intended to exclude or offend those who are blind from birth or who became blind later in life.

There is no universal definition of *vision impairment*. NASEM (2016) defines it as a measure of the functional limitation of one or both eyes or of other parts of the visual system that results from vision loss. The Centers for Disease Control and Prevention (CDC, n.d.-e) defines it as the inability to read letters on the 20/50 line or below on a Snellen eye chart with one's better eye.

Similar terms include *partial sight, partial blindness,* and *poor vision.* These are infrequently used.

THE SNELLEN EYE CHART

A Snellen eye chart (developed by Dutch ophthalmologist Herman Snellen in 1862) usually contains 11 lines of letters. The first line contains one large letter. Letters in each subsequent line are progressively smaller, with the bottom line containing the smallest letters of all.

The eye chart is used for eye tests. The person taking the eye test stands 20 feet from the chart and reads back the letters on each line of the chart. People who can read the 20/20 line of the chart from 20 feet away have "normal vision," which describes eyes without impairment. (More on the 20/20 line in a moment.) People who are unable to do so are said to have vision impairment. The lowest line they can read indicates the degree of vision impairment.

Each line on the chart is represented by a ratio called a *Snellen fraction*. The Snellen fraction for the top line of the chart is 20/200. This is because the letter on this line can be easily seen from 200 feet away by someone with normal vision, but only 20 feet by someone with a high level of vision impairment. A Snellen fraction of 20/50 indicates that the letters on the corresponding line can easily be seen from 50 feet away by someone with normal vision, but only 20 feet away by someone with vision impairment. And so on. Those who can read the 20/20 line of the Snellen chart correctly are said to have 20/20 vision.

The Snellen eye chart measures *visual acuity*. This describes the sharpness or clarity of vision. Visual acuity is assessed by one's ability to discern objects from a given distance according to a fixed standard. It reflects the distance between the eye and an object at which the object becomes blurry. There are slight differences in how vision loss measured with a Snellen eye chart is categorized. One general approach is as follows (WHO, 2019b):

- Mild vision loss/impairment or near-normal vision: 20/40 to 20/60

- Moderate vision loss/impairment or moderate low vision: 20/70 to 20/160

- Severe vision loss/impairment or severe low vision: 20/200 to 20/400

- Profound visual loss/impairment or profound low vision: 20/500 to 20/1000

- Near-total blindness/near-total vision loss/impairment: < 20/1000

- **Total blindness/total vision loss/impairment:** No light perception

Notice the use of the term "low vision" in the preceding bulleted list. This is another term to describe vision loss. *Low vision* is defined as visual impairment that is not correctable by standard eyeglasses, contact lenses, medications, or surgery, and that interferes with daily activities. This is more of a functional definition than one based on a measure of visual acuity using the Snellen eye chart. Low vision has been identified as the third most common reason in the US for impaired functioning in people 70 years of age and older (NEI, 2019b). Age by itself does not cause low vision, however. It is caused by other diseases associated with aging. The NEI (2019b) estimates that low vision affects more than 3 million Americans age 40 and older, and its prevalence is projected to increase over time.

> Low vision ranks below only arthritis and heart disease as the reason for impaired daily functioning in Americans over the age of 70.

Dillon, Gu, Hoffman, and Ko (2010) define *blindness* as severe visual impairment that cannot be corrected by standard glasses, contact lenses, medicine, or surgery. *Total blindness* refers to complete loss of sight, including light perception. Relatively few (15%) of those with vision loss have complete loss of light perception in which even light perception is absent (American Foundation for the Blind, n.d.)

There is a difference between total blindness and legal blindness. In the US, *legal blindness* describes when vision in the better eye is 20/200 even with the best correction; WHO defines legal blindness as 20/400 in the better eye (WHO, 2019b). The definition of legal blindness is used to determine eligibility for vocational training, re-habilitation, schooling, disability benefits, assistive devices, and tax exemptions.

A newer definition of legal blindness relies on the results of as-sessments that use a specialized low vision eye chart that measures visual acuity between 20/100 and 20/200 or a constricted visual field in the better-seeing eye. *Visual field* refers to the total area an individual can see to the side when looking straight ahead. It describes the "window" of each eye through which people see the environment around them. A decreased visual field results in a partial or total "closure" of this window. This is a major determinant of legal blindness and, often, one's eligibility to obtain a driver's license.

Rather than focusing solely on the results of various eye exams, it's useful to consider the effects of vision loss on a person's ability to function in the environment:

- **Mild vision loss:** With mild vision loss (20/40 to 20/60), people may not be able to read street signs, recognize people or objects across a room, read books and newspapers with regular-size print, view computer or television screens, distinguish between denominations of paper money, or read food-packaging labels, receipts, or medication directions.

- **Moderate vision loss:** With moderate vision loss (20/70 to 20/160), additional limitations may affect people's ability to recognize faces, read highway signs or large-print documents, write checks or complete forms, drive safely, and walk in unfamiliar locations, especially at dusk.

- **Severe vision loss:** Those with severe vision loss (20/200 to 20/400) may be unable to read large-print text or walk safely.

- **Profound vision loss:** People with profound vision loss (20/500 to 20/1000) may be limited to seeing shapes only. They might be unable to shave or apply makeup or to shop or cook. They might also rely on audio input (e.g., audiobooks) rather than visual input (e.g., print books).

- **Near-total or total vision loss:** People with near-total (<20/1000) or total vision loss (no light perception) receive little if any visual input and must rely on others or on assistive devices to navigate the environment (NASEM, 2016).

The effects of various levels of vision loss on one's ability to carry out specific tasks or functions will depend on that person's overall level of function and on the importance of these specific activities to the individual.

PREVALENCE OF VISION LOSS

WHO (2019b) estimates that at least 2.6 billion people around the world have vision impairment or blindness. Of these, at least 1 billion have a vision impairment that could have been prevented or has yet to be addressed. As with many disabilities, underserved populations and low- and middle-income countries are affected more than high-income countries and those where people have ready access to healthcare. People at particular risk for untreated vision impairment are women, migrants, indigenous people, and those living in rural communities. WHO (2019b) predicts that due to the growth and aging of the global population, behavioral and lifestyle issues, and urbanization, the number of people with eye conditions, vision impairment, and blindness will increase in the coming decades.

The CDC (n.d.-c) estimates that approximately 14 million people in the US over 12 years of age have vision impairment, including 1.02 million people who are blind. Between 8.2 and 11 million people have vision impairment due to undiagnosed or uncorrected refractive error (URE). Other estimates of prevalence are even higher (NASEM, 2016).

Refractive error describes when the shape of the eye hinders its ability to focus accurately. The most common types of refractive error are near-sightedness (myopia), in which faraway objects seem blurry, far-sightedness (hyperopia and presbyopia), in which close objects seem blurry, and astigmatism (all objects regardless of distance seem blurry). Hyperopia and presbyopia have similar effects, but their underlying causes differ.

Blindness or impaired vision is among the 10 most frequent disabilities of adults ages 18 and older in the US. For both men and women, non-Hispanic white people in the US have the highest prevalence of vision loss.

The CDC (n.d.-c) estimates that 6.8% of US children 18 years of age or younger have a diagnosis of eye and vision disorders, with 3% of children younger than 18 blind or visually impaired—that is, they have difficulty seeing even with glasses or contact lenses.

According to the CDC (n.d.-c), by 2050, the number of people with vision impairment of 20/200 or worse will double to approximately 2.01 million, 6.95 million people will have vision impairment even with best correction, and 16.4 million will have vision impairment due to URE. These increases will be due to the rapidly aging population, and to the growing population of people with diabetes (CDC, n.d.-c).

Vision loss in the US and around world should be considered a public health issue (WHO, 2019b) for the following reasons (CDC, n.d.-d):

- Its effects on a large number of people

- The resulting disability and decreased quality of life

- High costs to people, communities, and countries

- Its predicted increasing prevalence over the next 30 years

- Its perception as a threat

- The need for community- or population-level interventions

The CDC (n.d.-d) reports that 80% of people with vision loss could improve their vision through refractive correction (prescription glasses or contact lenses).

However, this issue does not receive adequate attention in the public health arena.

CAUSES OF VISION LOSS

To understand vision loss, it helps to understand how vision works:

1. Light enters the eye through the cornea.

2. The light passes through the aqueous humor, pupil lens, and vitreous humor to the retina.

3. Light-sensitive tissues, or *photoreceptors*, called rods and cones in the retina convert the light into neural impulses.

4. The neural impulses pass through the optic nerves to the thalamus and then to the brain's cerebral cortex, where they are interpreted as recognizable images.

The various physical structures of the eye must be intact and functioning properly to focus the light on the retina, to convert it to neural impulses, and to transmit the impulses through the optic nerves to the brain (NASEM, 2016). Damage or dysfunction in any part of the system can result in vision impairment, low vision, or blindness.

Vision loss can be due to disorders or changes that affect any one of the many structures or functions of the eye or brain that affect sight (NASEM, 2016). These include the following:

- **Lens:** Damage to the lens results in cataracts and refractive errors.

- **Anterior chamber:** Damage to the anterior chamber results in glaucoma.

- **Cornea:** Abrasion or damage to cornea can occur with corneal scarring due to measles and vitamin A deficiency disorders.

- **Vitreous humor:** Vitreous hemorrhages can result in impaired vision, "floaters," and other eye conditions.

- **Pupil:** Damage to the pupil is often due to penetrating eye injury.

- **Retina:** Conditions like diabetes can damage the retina and affect vision. Other retinal conditions that affect vision include retinopathy, retinal detachment, macular degeneration, retinitis pigmentosa, and retinopathy of prematurity.

Another major cause of vision loss is aging. Neurological disorders can also affect vision. For example, strokes can cause a variety of vision changes, and multiple sclerosis can affect the optic nerve, which causes vision loss. Vision loss after traumatic brain injury is also common, although its diagnosis is often delayed.

Congenital vision loss and blindness present at birth or soon thereafter can occur due to maternal infection, genetics, prematurity, vitamin deficiency, congenital abnormalities, and lesions of the optic nerve and higher visual pathways. Differences in causes of childhood vision impairment and blindness are seen in high-income countries versus low-income countries.

The process by which eyesight deteriorates varies. In many cases, decreases in vision are gradual. People experiencing vision loss might not even notice it until their inability to see begins to affect everyday activities. However, sudden vision loss can also occur. This is generally considered an emergency requiring immediate attention to prevent permanent loss of vision.

Vision loss is often chronic, progressive, and irreversible.

CONSEQUENCES OF VISION LOSS

Vision loss or blindness has serious consequences throughout one's life if treatment and supportive services are not available or not provided. With inadequate access to quality eye care and provision of proper glasses or contact lenses, even mild or moderate vision impairment can have a significant effect on an individual's cognitive, social, and economic well-being. Vision loss and blindness in children can result in delayed development of motor, language, emotional, social, and cognitive skills (WHO, 2019b). Uncorrected vision loss in school-age children can affect their learning, education, and self-esteem. Their educational achievement is threatened, which has lifelong consequences for them, their families, and society as a whole. Their future participation in the workforce is also affected, with lower levels of employment or underemployment a possible outcome.

Vision loss in adults can interfere with education, work, and independence, as well as the ability to obtain healthcare and to maintain health (WHO, 2019b). The more severe the vision impairment, the greater its impact (NASEM, 2016).

Although many adults with significant vision loss or blindness live productive, healthy lives, others do not. Some have difficulty maintaining their health and quality of life. Many adults with vision loss or blindness experience unemployment or underemployment and higher rates of depression and anxiety than the general population. Vision loss also affects their ability to read, drive, prepare meals, watch television, and attend to personal affairs. Severe vision loss increases the risk of violence and abuse, bullying, and sexual violence, as well as motor vehicle crashes. Finally, because vision aids us in navigating three-dimensional space, walking and using stairs become increasingly difficult with vision loss. This results in increased risk of falls and subsequent fractures, particularly hip fractures (NASEM, 2016).

Self-care becomes more difficult with vision loss, as does managing other health issues. People with vision loss who have chronic diseases such as diabetes, hypertension, heart disease, and stroke have higher mortality compared to those with chronic diseases and no vision impairment. On a related note, people with vision impairment due to diabetes may have difficulty conducting foot checks, preparing and eating nutritious meals, taking the correct doses of medication, and obtaining medication refills. This puts them at increased risk of further deterioration in vision due to persistent hyperglycemia, failing to notice changes in their feet that require the attention of a healthcare provider, and medication errors (CDC, n.d.-d; NASEM, 2016; WHO, 2019a).

Vision loss is particularly detrimental to older adults. In addition to causing social isolation, family stress, and poor quality of life, vision loss or blindness in aging adults may limit their mobility, affect their cognitive status, and make rehabilitation efforts less effective. Older adults with vision loss are also more likely to enter a nursing home earlier than others and are at greater risk of developing other health conditions or dying prematurely.

According to WHO (2019b), people who live long enough will have at least one eye condition during their lifetime. Although most of these conditions will not cause severe vision loss or blindness, those that can do so must be treated to prevent vision loss.

People with significant vision loss often rely on support from caregivers such as family members, friends, and others. These caregivers may be responsible for assisting with activities of daily living (e.g., shopping, preparing food, maintaining a household, managing family finances), self-care (e.g., hygiene, health-related activities such as preparing medications), and transportation (e.g., driving the affected family member to healthcare visits). They might also be called on to assist with physical care as well as emotional and social support.

Vision loss and blindness can also have a major impact on the economic status of people, families, and society as a whole because of direct medical expenses as well as indirect expenses that result from loss of mobility and productivity. Experts estimate that in 2013, these direct and indirect expenses in the US exceeded $140 billion (CDC, n.d.-d). Family members who provide assistance, care, and support for someone with vision loss might also experience an adverse economic impact—especially if performing these tasks requires them to withdraw from the workforce.

CHARACTERISTICS OF VISION LOSS

Many disorders that occur across the life span, from birth to old age, can cause vision loss, blindness, and resulting disability. These include the following:

- Hereditary and genetic factors

- The aging process

- Chronic disorders that affect vision (e.g., diabetes and hypertension)

- Uncorrected refractive errors

- Eye injury

- Brain injury

- Infectious and congenital issues that affect infants and children

Table 8.1 describes characteristics of select causes of vision loss and blindness. The causes listed here represent but do not include all possible causes of vision loss and blindness.

TABLE 8.1   CHARACTERISTICS OF SELECT TYPES OF DISORDERS CAUSING VISION LOSS

COMMON CAUSES OF VISION LOSS	CHARACTERISTICS
UNCORRECTED REFRACTIVE ERROR (URE)	
The leading cause of vision impairment in the US and worldwide. It has only recently been identified as a cause of blindness. Worldwide, 145 million people have significant distance visual impairment, and 8 million are blind due to URE (Holden, 2007). Recent studies in the US indicate that proper refractive correction could improve vision among 11 million Americans ages 12 and older (NEI, 2019a).	There are different types of refractive errors: • **Myopia:** Near-sightedness • **Hyperopia:** Far-sightedness • **Astigmatism:** Distorted vision at all distances • **Presbyopia:** Aging-related loss of the ability to focus up close—e.g., to read letters and numbers in a phone book; need to hold newspaper farther away to see clearly; occurs between age 40 and 50

continues

TABLE 8.1 CHARACTERISTICS OF SELECT TYPES OF DISORDERS CAUSING VISION LOSS (CONT.)

COMMON CAUSES OF VISION LOSS	CHARACTERISTICS
UNCORRECTED REFRACTIVE ERROR (URE) (CONT.)	
Risk factors for URE include the following: • Low socioeconomic status • Poor access to healthcare, including eye assessments • Genetics, a nonmodifiable risk factor	These refractive errors can be corrected by eyeglasses, contact lenses, or in some cases surgery. As many as 72% of people in the US with vision loss and 20% of those with blindness could experience clinical improvement with vision screening and proper refractive correction.
DIABETIC RETINOPATHY	
A microvascular complication of diabetes that affects the retina and blood vessels of the eye, causing microaneurysms. These lesions are the most common characteristic of diabetic retinopathy. Other effects are retinal detachment, preretinal or vitreous hemorrhage, glaucoma, macular edema, and capillary nonperfusion (Zhang et al., 2010). Risk factors for diabetic retinopathy include the following (Diabetes Prevention Program Research Group, 2007): • Long duration of diabetes • Hyperglycemia • Hypertension • Dyslipidemia This condition is more likely to occur in men, non-Hispanic Blacks, and those of Mexican American heritage (Zhang et al., 2010).	Diabetic retinopathy may be asymptomatic in the early stages, even as symptoms progress. Thus, frequent dilated eye exams are essential for early detection. Later symptoms include the following: • Difficulty reading or clearly seeing faraway objects • Blurred vision • Floating spots, blind spots, or streaks in the field of vision • Blindness Preventive measure: • Control of systemic blood glucose level Treatments include the following (NEI, 2019a): • Laser treatment for growth of new blood vessels • Eye injections of anti-VEGF agents to control macular edema • Corticosteroids According to the CDC (n.d.-c), 90% of cases of blindness caused by diabetes are preventable.

AGE-RELATED MACULAR DEGENERATION (AMD)

A degenerative eye disorder associated with aging that results in the breakdown of the light-sensitive cells in the macula (the part of the retina that enables the eye to see fine details). AMD affects 1.8 million people in the US who are age 40 and older and is the leading cause of permanent impairment of reading and fine or close-up vision among people age 65 years and older. Experts estimate that by 2050 the number of US adults over 50 years of age with AMD will be 5.44 million.

Smoking has been identified as a modifiable risk factor for AMD (NASEM, 2016).

In the early and intermediate stages of AMD, changes in vision may not be noticeable without a dilated eye examination, despite ongoing damage to structures of the visual system. AMD causes blurred central vision needed for reading and driving. AMD may also result in difficulty recognizing faces. The need for more light to read and perform other tasks may arise. AMD is largely untreatable, although promising treatments include nutritional therapies and certain injections.

CATARACTS

The clouding or discoloration of the lens of the eye, which makes it difficult to see. Cataracts are the leading cause of blindness worldwide and of vision loss in the US. More than 20.5 million (17.2%) people in the US over 40 years of age have a cataract in one or both eyes.

Risk factors include the following:

- Eye trauma
- Eye surgery
- Exposure to ultraviolet (UV) radiation
- Aging
- Smoking

Cataracts can occur at any age. Children can be born with cataracts.

Treatments include the removal and possible replacement of the affected lens. The use of eyeglasses, magnifying glasses, and better lighting may help reduce symptoms (NEI, 2019b).

continues

TABLE 8.1 CHARACTERISTICS OF SELECT TYPES OF DISORDERS CAUSING VISION LOSS (CONT.)

COMMON CAUSES OF VISION LOSS	CHARACTERISTICS
GLAUCOMA (OPEN ANGLE)	
A group of diseases that can cause vision loss and blindness due to fluid buildup in the anterior chamber of the eye and increased intraocular pressure (IOP) that damages the optic nerve over time. Primary open-angle glaucoma is the most common type in the US, affecting 3 million people. It is the second leading cause of blindness worldwide (CDC, n.d.-b). Risk factors include the following: • Older than 60 years of age • African American or Hispanic/Latinx and older than 40 years of age • Family history The following increase the risk of glaucoma: • Eye injury • Eye surgery • The use of steroid medications (in some people) In addition, diabetes doubles the risk of developing glaucoma (CDC, n.d.-b).	Early in the course of the disease, vision remains normal. Thus, regular dilated eye exams are necessary to detect glaucoma. If untreated, peripheral vision slowly deteriorates, with narrowing of the visual field. This may be described as looking through a dark tunnel. Loss of central vision occurs, with progression to blindness. Treatments include the following: • Control of eye pressure through therapeutic eye drops • Oral medication • Laser surgery
EYE INJURY	
A leading cause of blindness in children (National Eye Institute [NEI] & National Eye Health Education Program Institutes of Health, 2016). More than 2.5 million eye injuries occur in the US each year, resulting in nearly 50,000 people permanently losing part or all of their vision.	Risk of eye injury can be reduced with the use of protective eyewear when engaging in activities (such as sports) or in environments (such as construction sites) known to be associated with eye injury.

VISION LOSS AND BLINDNESS IN CHILDREN

Defined as difficulty seeing despite use of glasses or contact lenses. Vision loss and blindness affect 3% of children. Disability due to vision loss and blindness is one of the most common types of disability among children (CDC, n.d.-a).

More than half of affected children have one or more developmental disabilities. This increases the likelihood that vision loss will not be adequately addressed. (CDC, n.d.-a).

Retinopathy of prematurity (ROP) is common with preterm birth and can lead to lifelong vision impairment and blindness. The smaller a baby is at birth, the more likely that baby is to develop ROP (Kim, Port, Swan, Campbell, Chan, & Chiang, (2018).

The effects of vision loss and blindness in young children are substantial, potentially affecting the development of motor, language, emotional, social, and cognitive skills (WHO, 2019b). Uncorrected vision loss in school-age children can affect their learning, education, and self-esteem.

DEAF-BLINDNESS

People can be both deaf and blind—losing both their hearing and their vision. There is great variability in the severity of deaf-blindness. This variability depends on the underlying cause of deaf-blindness and the age of onset. Because people rely heavily on both hearing and vision to navigate the world, severe cases of deaf-blindness can greatly limit communication, education, employment, and independence.

Experts have identified more than 70 causes of deaf-blindness. These include hereditary disorders, disorders that occur because of circumstances at birth (e.g., preterm birth), and disorders that occur later in life—after the individual has developed speech and language skills. People can be born deaf-blind if their mother contracted an infection (such as rubella, Zika virus, or cytomegalovirus) while pregnant. Age-related issues can also cause deaf-blindness.

Most children who are deaf-blind have some usable vision, usable hearing, or both, but typically nowhere near what their sighted and hearing peers have.

A sizable percent of the population of children who are deaf-blind also have other disabilities, including cognitive and physical disabilities. They may also have complex health needs or behavioral challenges (National Center on Deaf-Blindness, 2007).

People who are deaf-blind are likely to have limited or no access to information that is available to others. This can lead to dependence, lack of social interaction, and other issues that affect their ability to live and thrive in the world. It is worth noting, however, that people who are deaf-blind have graduated from law school, become authors and actors, and succeeded in many other fields. Still, most people who experience deaf-blindness require accommodations to access the world around them and lead independent lives.

Healthcare professionals generally lack sensitivity to and knowledge about the health-related needs of people with vision or hearing loss. They are even less aware of the needs of people who have deaf-blindness. Being deaf-blind typically presents a major barrier to access to healthcare. Although the Americans with Disabilities Act (ADA) has mandated that healthcare providers provide reasonable accommodations for all people with disability, including those who are deaf-blind, healthcare professionals have received little education or training to prepare them to do so (Withers & Speight, 2017). It is important for healthcare professionals to understand how vision and hearing loss, and the combination of the two, impact the lives of those affected so that necessary accommodations can be put in place to provide the greatest degree of access. They must also be aware of strategies and aids that can be used to communicate with people who are deaf-blind, such as Teletouch devices, sighted guides, guide dogs, and others. For more information about communication strategies, watch the video "Communicating with Deaf Blind People" (https://www.youtube.com/watch?v=usaf3bVVvjY).

CARING FOR PEOPLE WITH DISABILITY DUE TO VISION LOSS

Like hearing loss, vision loss (including low vision, vision impairment, and blindness) is often invisible to others. This is because many people with significant vision loss do not use assistive devices such as canes, guides, or service dogs, or show other outward signs of vision loss.

Vision loss is "invisible" in another way. Because it often occurs gradually, it may not become obvious to people until it begins to interfere with usual activities, including family and social life or employment. So, people may be unaware of the magnitude of their vision loss and of available resources that could improve their lives.

The fact that a high percentage of people with vision loss could have their vision improved through treatment (such as prescription glasses or contact lenses) but have not sought or received such treatment suggests that healthcare for this population should include discussions of these issues. On a related note, nurses should treat someone whose vision loss or blindness *is known* but who is seeking healthcare for a health issue not related to vision as a person who happens to have vision loss or blindness rather than as a "blind person." In other words, treat the patient as a person first.

People with vision loss or blindness encounter various barriers in their efforts to obtain safe, effective, timely, and patient-centered healthcare (O'Day, Killeen, & Iezzoni, 2004). These include barriers to appropriate eye or vision care as well as barriers to healthcare in general. One study identified four categories of such barriers (O'Day et al., 2004):

- Lack of respect on the part of healthcare providers, including the assumption that people with vision loss or blindness cannot participate in their own care

- Communication barriers

- Physical access barriers

- Information barriers (e.g., receiving written materials in small text rather than in large print or in Braille or in audio form)

People with eye conditions that result in vision impairment or blindness who face environmental or physical access barriers may experience limitations in everyday functioning.

Harrison, Mackert, and Watkins (2010) report the following assumptions and biases of healthcare providers toward people who are blind:

- They cannot take care of themselves and need a caretaker.

- They have no cognitive skills.

- They rely on government assistance.

- Their intelligence and ability to explain what they need are unreliable.

- They can or need to be treated differently from others seeking healthcare.

Healthcare professionals often lack knowledge about vision loss. They tend to underestimate the prevalence of vision loss in the population; the effects of vision loss on people's everyday lives, health, and healthcare; and the importance of providing information in accessible formats. Healthcare professionals also tend to overestimate their ability to meet and support the needs of people with vision loss.

Healthcare providers are often uncomfortable talking to people with vision loss or blindness.

There is also widespread lack of awareness among healthcare professionals of effective ways to interact with people with vision loss or blindness (NASEM, 2016). That is, they use only conversation and written materials to communicate with people with vision loss and are unfamiliar with the need for other communication formats or strategies to tailor communication to people who have vision loss. These include the following:

- Identify and honor the communication preferences of the person who has vision loss or blindness.

- Note the person's communication preferences for subsequent interactions and for others.

- Face the person directly and at eye level.

- Gain the person's attention by speaking the individual's name first.

- Introduce yourself by name and explain your role and the reason for your presence, in good light.

- Direct all conversation to the person, not to a caregiver or companion.

- Use a conversational tone of voice. Shouting or raising your voice will *not* make conversation easier to follow. Indeed, it may make it more difficult.

- If more than one person is in the room or engaged in a group conversation, make it clear who you are and to whom you are speaking.

- Avoid nodding and shaking your head. Use verbal responses instead.

- Explain what is going on around the person, what you are doing and why, and what is expected of the person.

- Orient the person to the environment—the parameters of the room, the location of doors and objects, and so on.

- If you need to touch the person—for example, to take his or her blood pressure or temperature—warn the person ahead of time, explain what you are about to do, and describe what sensation the person will feel or experience.

- When you are moving away or leaving the room or site, inform the person and note when you will return.

- Ask the person what method of recording conversation, directions, or instructions would be most useful (e.g., audio recording, Braille, large-print writing, other).

- Provide educational materials, such as preoperative or preprocedural instructions or reminders, in large print (for people who can read it) or Braille.

- Use assistive technology (e.g., videos or pamphlets with large print, or audio recordings) when communicating.

- Don't just hand over printed material. Go over it with the person.

- Periodically verify with the person that you are being clear in your conversation and explanation.

- Determine whether guidance or support is required.

- Ask if the person has any questions or would like any information repeated.

- Pay attention to the person's body language. A puzzled look or other gesture may indicate misunderstanding. Tactfully ask if the person understood you or ask leading questions so you know your message got across.

- If the person uses an aid or assistive device, make sure the individual has access to it before you leave.

There are many assistive and adaptive devices to aid people with low vision. The most common of these are prescription glasses (spectacles) and contact lenses. Several other optical devices assist people with low vision by magnifying objects, such as magnifying glasses, hand-held or stand-mounted magnifiers, and telescopes to see more distant objects.

Advances in technology have resulted in many more assistive devices, including smartphone apps that can be used by individuals with low vision. However, it is important to ensure that these individuals have these devices with them when they interact with healthcare providers. It is equally important for healthcare providers to take the time to enable individuals with low vision to use these devices.

> People who have eyeglasses and other assistive devices should be encouraged or reminded to use them to make vision and communication easier.

Accommodations that can be used to provide information for people with vision impairment and blindness include:

- Written materials in large print or Braille, depending on the individual's needs

- Videos to illustrate and describe surgeries and other medical procedures, if the person has some vision
- Closed circuit TV (CCTV) magnifiers to magnify video
- Screen reader apps for computers, smartphones, and tablets to convert text to speech
- Audio and electronic books

The electronic devices listed here are becoming increasingly available for use by people with vision loss. However, there can be considerable expense associated with the purchase of some of these devices.

Healthcare providers would benefit from learning how to use these accommodations—or to at least understand how those who use them navigate through content.

One area that is lagging in accommodations is the internet. Although some healthcare providers assume that all information available on the internet can be accessed and understood by those with visual impairment and blindness, few websites have been made accessible to make them useful for all. That said, guides for increasing the accessibility of websites for individuals with visual impairment do exist and can be used by individuals and organizations to make their websites more accessible.

Other devices to assist people with visual impairment include those with audible signals to alert them of the time and about measures—for example, from blood pressure and blood glucose testing.

There have been many recent advances in development of assistive devices and navigational aids for people with vision loss or blindness. These include smartphone apps that read street signs and convert medication labels to text, robotic walking canes, and others. Haptic devices use sensors and vibration to indicate the presence of nearby objects, which increases the independence of individuals with vision loss. In addition, recent advances in biotechnology have seen the first in-human trials—and in some cases market approval—of stem cell and gene therapies as well as retinal prostheses to treat vision loss and blindness. These and other advancements hold promise for people with vision loss and blindness. However, there are complex engineering and biophysical obstacles still to be overcome (Bloch, Luo, & da Cruz, 2019).

> Despite advancements, the use of visual rehabilitation services and of visual adaptive devices among adults with visual impairment remains low.

Some people who have vision loss or are blind have service animals—usually dogs. Service dogs undergo considerable training to carry out tasks for their person (called a *handler*) and are considered working animals rather than pets. Service dogs are often critical in enabling people with significant vision loss to maintain independence and participate in society. The ADA mandates that service dogs be allowed to accompany their handler anywhere the public is allowed to go. As the use of service dogs increases, healthcare providers, regardless of setting, are likely to encounter them. Policies of healthcare settings (if such policies exist) should serve as useful guidelines with regard to service dogs (Krawczyk, 2016).

EDUCATING NURSES TO CARE FOR PEOPLE WITH DISABILITY DUE TO VISION LOSS

A number of strategies and resources are available for nurses and other healthcare professionals to increase their knowledge about vision loss and blindness. These include the following:

- Add content, modules, or courses on vision loss and blindness to existing curriculum components in classroom, simulation, home care, and clinical experiences.

- Assign students to view and write a report on one of the healthcare stories about people with vision loss and blindness, available from https://https://visionaware.org/emotional-support/personal-stories/.

- Assign students to read a story on the experience of a child with vision loss or blindness at https://www.brailleinstitute.org.

- Establish collaborative relationships with agencies or healthcare settings that provide care and services to people with vision loss and blindness for student placement (e.g., schools for the blind; centers for independent living; Community Center for the Blind and Visually Impaired).

- Initiate clinical sites for and with people with vision loss and blindness and their families for student clinical assignments and visits. (Provide education to students before first assignment to sites.)

- Identify community agencies with populations of people with vision loss or blindness to demonstrate for students the ability of people with such conditions to participate in activities, work, and school.

- Invite people with vision loss or blindness to participate in lectures and panel discussions to enable students to become comfortable asking about these conditions and to learn firsthand about the health-related experiences of people who have them (after ensuring that appropriate communication strategies are available).

- Explore inclusion of people with vision loss or blindness as standardized patients in simulations. Provide training so that expectations are clear to those with vision loss or blindness, faculty, staff, and students.

> Only people with vision loss or blindness should serve as standardized patients with vision loss or who are blind. This ensures authentic experiences and prevents stereotyping.

- Build on existing classroom, simulation, home care, and clinical experiences by adding case studies of people with vision loss or blindness.

- Model for students positive attitudes, behaviors, and skills that relate to people with vision loss or blindness.

- Use available resources to better teach students about disability due to vision loss or blindness (see the following sidebar).

- Assign students to identify modifications to patient teaching plans and strategies to accommodate people with varying types and severity of vision loss.

- Explore other campus resources, personnel, and faculty who have expertise/experience with people with vision loss.

- Participate in disability studies lectures, programs, or courses if available on university or college campus.

- Identify and collaborate with others on campus with a focus on people with disability (e.g., Disabilities Services, Student Services) to identify shared interests and provide mutual support.

- Become active in disability-related organizations in your city or state or on campus to increase visibility and recognition of the need to ensure that all people, including those with vision loss or blindness, receive appropriate education, healthcare, and services.

- Establish a relationship with people with vision loss or blindness in their own environment as well as in a healthcare setting to learn about their everyday issues, challenges, and accomplishments.

- Explore and develop your own creative and innovative approaches to addressing vision loss disability in curriculum. Focus on the day-to-day lives of those affected rather than limiting your focus to acute care issues in hospital settings.

- Initiate a classroom discussion on deaf-blindness, and on strategies for approaching people who have deaf-blindness, to determine how to address their healthcare needs.

RESOURCES TO TEACH HEALTHCARE PROVIDERS ABOUT VISION LOSS DISABILITY

- **American Association of the Deaf Blind (AADB) (http://aadb.org):** This website provides links to resources, FAQs, and fact sheets for people who are deaf-blind, their parents, and the general public.

- **American Foundation for the Blind (https://www.afb.org):** This website provides detailed descriptions of vision loss, low-vision optical and nonoptical devices, and advocacy efforts.

- **Communicating with Deaf-Blind People (https://www.youtube.com/watch?v=usaf3bVVvjY):** This video, available on YouTube, illustrates five communication strategies that can be used by healthcare clinicians and others to communicate with people who are deaf-blind.

- **Guide Dog Users, Inc. (GDUI) (https://guidedogusersinc.org):** This organization provides peer support, advocacy, information for guide-dog users, and links to legal resources. It also publishes a guide for guide-dog users to ensure that their rights are protected.

- **Helen Keller National Center for Deaf-Blind Youths and Adults (https://www.helenkeller.org/hknc/lesson/introduction-deaf-blindness):** This organization is named after Helen Keller, an American author, political activist, and public speaker, and the first deaf-blind person to earn a Bachelor of Arts degree. Its website provides a detailed explanation of deaf-blindness and features a quiz to test your knowledge.

- **National Family Association for Deaf-Blind (NFADB) (https://nfadb.org):** This organization raises up the voices of families of people who are deaf-blind and advocates for their unique needs. It provides support, connects families with other families, collaborates with other organizations at the state and national level, and advises professionals.

- **National Federation of the Blind (NFB) (https://www.nfb.org):** This website addresses advocacy efforts for people who are blind and provides links to many other resources.

SUMMARY

Most people with vision loss or blindness from early age have been evaluated and treated for these issues. However, many people who have developed vision loss over time have not. Healthcare professionals are likely to encounter both of these groups throughout the healthcare system. Therefore, all healthcare professionals need to be knowledgeable about vision loss and blindness (as well as deaf-blindness) and be prepared to use appropriate communication strategies. Nurses whose role involves preparing patients for surgery, diagnostic procedures, and hospital discharge must be proactive in obtaining and providing educational materials that are accessible to people with vision loss. Healthcare professionals who provide care for people with vision loss, blindness, and deaf-blindness must be prepared to address their immediate healthcare needs while also considering how vision impairment might affect their ability to obtain care and communicate with others. Healthcare professionals should also identify people with vision loss who have not been diagnosed as such and help guide them to receive effective treatment. Additionally, informing those with vision loss about advances in technology and referring them to sources that can aid in the selection of appropriate devices can be useful in increasing their independence.

REFERENCES

American Foundation for the Blind (n.d.) Low vision and legal blindness terms and descriptions. Retrieved from https://www.afb.org/blindness-and-low-vision/eye-conditions/low-vision-and-legal-blindness-terms-and-descriptions?gclid=CjwKCAjw1ej5BRBhEiwAfHyh1OkVdcBFElByXmMo5s1fCAVhlMcn-UJcDJND-4K-0nAytgf-KxhhixoCrI8QAvD_BwE

Bloch, E., Luo, Y., & da Cruz, L. (2019). Advances in retinal prosthesis systems. *Therapeutic Advances in Ophthalmology, 11*, 1–16. doi:10.1177/2515841418817501

Centers for Disease Control and Prevention. (n.d.-a). Basics of vision and eye health. Retrieved from https://www.cdc.gov/visionhealth/basics/index.html

Centers for Disease Control and Prevention. (n.d.-b). Don't let glaucoma steal your sight! Retrieved from https://www.cdc.gov/features/glaucoma-awareness/index.html

Centers for Disease Control and Prevention. (n.d.-c). Improving the nation's vision health. Retrieved from https://www.cdc.gov/visionhealth/pdf/vhi.pdf

Centers for Disease Control and Prevention. (n.d.-d). Vision and eye health toolkit. Retrieved from https://www.cdc.gov/visionhealth/programs/vision-eye-health-tool.html

Centers for Disease Control and Prevention. (n.d.-e). Vision impairment and blindness. Retrieved from https://www.cdc.gov/visionhealth/vehss/data/studies/vision-impairment-and-blindness.html

Diabetes Prevention Program Research Group. (2007). The prevalence of retinopathy in impaired glucose tolerance and recent-onset diabetes in the Diabetes Prevention Program. *Diabetic Medicine, 24*(2), 137–144. doi:10.1111/j.1464-5491.2007.02043.x

Dillon, C. F., Gu, Q., Hoffman, H. J., & Ko, C. (2010). Vision, hearing, balance, and sensory impairment in Americans aged 70 years and over: United States, 1999–2006. NCHS Data Brief No. 31. Retrieved from https://www.cdc.gov/nchs/products/databriefs/db31.htm

Harrison, T. C., Mackert, M., & Watkins, C. (2010). A qualitative analysis of health literacy issues among women with visual impairments. *Research in Gerontological Nursing, 3*(1), 49–60. doi:10.3928/19404921-20090731-01

Holden, B. A. (2007). Uncorrected refractive error: The major and most easily avoidable cause of vision loss. *Community Eye Health Journal, 20*(63), 37–39.

Kim, S. J., Port, A. D., Swan, R., Campbell, J. P., Chan, R. V. P., & Chiang, M. F. (2018). Retinopathy of prematurity: A review of risk factors and their clinical significance. *Survey of Ophthalmology, 63*(5), 618–637. doi:10.1016/j.survophthal.2018.04.002

Krawczyk, M. (2016). Caring for patients with service dogs: Information for healthcare providers. *Online Journal of Issues in Nursing, 22*(1), 7. doi:10.3912/OJIN.Vol22No01PPT45

National Academies of Sciences, Engineering, and Medicine. (2016). *Making eye health a population health imperative: Vision for tomorrow.* Washington, D.C.: The National Academies Press.

National Center on Deaf-Blindness. (2007). Children who are deaf-blind. Retrieved from https://www.nationaldb.org/info-center/children-who-are-practice-perspective

National Eye Institute. (2019a). Injections to treat diabetic retinopathy and diabetic macular edema. Retrieved from https://www.nei.nih.gov/learn-about-eye-health/eye-conditions-and-diseases/diabetic-retinopathy/injections-treat-diabetic-retinopathy-and-diabetic-macular-edema

National Eye Institute. (2019b). Low vision. Retrieved from https://www.nei.nih.gov/learn-about-eye-health/eye-conditions-and-diseases/low-vision

National Eye Institute & National Eye Health Education Program. (2016). National Health Education Program: Five-year agenda | 2012–2017. Retrieved from https://www.nei.nih.gov/sites/default/files/nehep-pdfs/NEHEP_Five-Year_Agenda_2012-2017.pdf

O'Day, B. L., Killeen, M., & Iezzoni, L. I. (2004). Improving health care experiences of persons who are blind or have low vision: Suggestions from focus groups. *American Journal of Medical Quality, 19*(5), 193–200. doi:10.1177/106286060401900503

Withers, J., & Speight, C. (2017). Health care for individuals with hearing loss or vision loss: A minefield of barriers to accessibility. *North Carolina Medical Journal, 78*(2), 107–112. Doi:10.18043/ncm.78.2.107

World Health Organization. (2019a). Blindness and vision impairment. Retrieved from https://www.who.int/news-room/fact-sheets/detail/blindness-and-visual-impairment

World Health Organization. (2019b). World report on vision. Retrieved from https://www.who.int/publications-detail/world-report-on-vision

Zhang, X., Saaddine, J. B., Chou, C. F., Cotch, M. F., Cheng, Y. J., Geiss, L. S., ... Klein, R. (2010). Prevalence of diabetic retinopathy in the United States, 2005–2008. *Journal of the American Medical Association*, 30(6), 649–656. doi:10.1001/jama.2010.1111

9

INCLUSION OF STUDENTS WITH DISABILITY: REDEFINING NURSING EDUCATION

–BETH MARKS, PHD, RN, FAAN
RESEARCH ASSOCIATE PROFESSOR
DEPARTMENT OF DISABILITY AND HUMAN DEVELOPMENT,
UNIVERSITY OF ILLINOIS AT CHICAGO

INTRODUCTION

Students with disability represent an untapped resource to redefine nursing education and practice. This chapter describes how key disability legislation and activism in the US has supported the emergence of new expectations, creative potential, and disability pride among students with disability and discusses how these changes intersect with nursing education and practice. The chapter illustrates the "what" of nursing education along with how nurses with disability can enhance culturally competent care. It also discusses ways in which students and nurses with disability can promote new and innovative "ways of knowing" to enhance patient care, lead the nursing profession in new directions, and improve health services. Finally, it presents and discusses a framework to expand diversity.

BACKGROUND: THE IMPETUS FOR CHANGE IN NURSING EDUCATION

People with disability represent the largest minority group in the US. Increasingly more people live with disability (US Census Bureau, 2012). With advances in healthcare and medicine, disability rights activism, and disability legislation that promotes the rights of people with disability, more individuals with disability are attending school, working in meaningful jobs, and considering careers in the health professions—including nursing.

About one in four Americans has a disability of some kind (US Census Bureau, 2012). While one typically thinks of a person with a disability as someone who uses a wheelchair or some other assistive device, more than 90% of disabilities are nonapparent to others (Steinmetz, 2006). Today, increasing numbers of students with disability are entering the postsecondary educational system due to the following societal shifts (US Department of Education Office of Civil Rights, 2011):

- Increased public awareness of legal protections and career options for people with disability

- Improved services and preparation in grades K–12
- Technology that bridges communication and accessibility gaps
- Veterans returning from deployments with disability ranging from traumatic brain injury, to post-traumatic stress disorder, to amputations

With more students and veterans who have a variety of disabilities seeking admission to nursing schools, an opportunity exists to bring different views and perspectives into nursing education and practice. The percentage of undergraduate students with a disability increased from 3% in 1978 to 20% in 2015 (Institute of Education Sciences [IES] National Center for Education Statistics, 2019; National Council on Disability, 2003). During this period, landmark civil rights laws pertaining to disability were passed, including the following:

- Section 504 of the 1973 Rehabilitation Act (Public Law 94-142)
- Education for All Handicapped Children Act (Public Law 94-142) in 1975
- The Americans with Disabilities Act (ADA) of 1990 (Public Law 101-336)
- The ADA Amendments Act of 2008 (Public Law 110-325)
- Section 503 of the Rehabilitation Act of 1973, as amended at 41 CFR Part 60-741, passed September 24, 2013 and effective on March 24, 2014: Federal Contract Compliance Programs (OFCCP) 7% rule requiring a national utilization goal to recruit, hire, promote, and retain individuals with disability

The percentages of undergraduate students with disability vary by characteristics such as veteran status, age, dependency status, and race/ethnicity. For example, disability is higher among undergraduate veterans (26%) than undergraduates who were not veterans (19%), higher among people age 30 and over (23%) than among people age 15 to 23 (18%), lower among Asian undergraduates (15%) compared to white, Hispanic, and Black students (21%, 18%, and 17%, respectively), and lower among postbaccalaureate students (12%) than undergraduates (19%) (IES National Center for Education Statistics, 2019).

Dr. Lisa Iezzoni, a physician with a disability, has identified several benefits of increasing the number of health professionals who identify as "disabled" to proactively confront disability-related barriers affecting patients (Iezzoni, 2016). Nursing students with disability can bring a wealth of knowledge about and experience in achieving goals through accommodations that could benefit patients with and without disability while also diversifying the health professions (Waliany, 2016). Nurses with disability who understand the many ingrained and erroneous assumptions about the daily lives, values, and expectations of persons with disability can challenge stigmatizing views and provide culturally and linguistically relevant care.

Faculty frequently ask, "Do people who do not meet the traditional requirements of an academic program, such as students with disability, have a place in nursing?" (Marks, 2007). A more relevant question may be, "How can we recruit, retain, matriculate, and graduate students with disability with diverse skill sets to become nurses who practice in a variety of settings?" Considering the needs to address contemporary health policy and workforce-development issues, educators might also consider asking the following questions:

- "What do people with disability bring to healthcare delivery, health policy, and patient outcomes?"

- "How can we provide an educational program that creates an accepting environment for students with disability?"

With new expectations for diversity in nursing education and practice, students with disability can bring innovative competencies and solutions in a dynamic nursing practice.

Responses to these questions will enhance learning spaces for all students and innovate new nursing practices.

DISABILITY IN NURSING EDUCATION: CHANGING LIVES

A disability experience—whether temporary or permanent—can happen to anyone, at any time, regardless of age, gender, race, or ethnicity. Whether someone is born with a disability or acquires one, nurses worldwide are among the first healthcare professionals to interact with people experiencing disability, along with their families and supports. As a result, nurses have a tremendous opportunity to change the life course for many people with disability.

People with disability often do not share their disability status with their family members (Bogart, 2020). Therefore, promoting nurse-patient concordance may have a positive effect among those who prefer it (Schnittker & Liang, 2006; Forber-Pratt, Lyew, Mueller, & Samples (2017). Research has documented the impact of perceived personal similarity with healthcare providers with higher ratings of trust, satisfaction, and intention to adhere to treatment recommendations (Street, O'Malley, Cooper, & Haidet, 2008).

As frontline healthcare professionals, nurses are critical in promoting patients' aspirations and goals. Nursing services are directly linked to quality and cost-effectiveness (American Nurses Association, 2020). Moreover, nurses have been voted the most trusted profession for the past 18 years (Reinhart, 2020). The positive values held by the public positions nurses to help people with disability integrate their disability within their sense of self. For example, consider what might happen when a nurse who uses a wheelchair rolls into the hospital room of a young girl diagnosed with cerebral palsy who is also a wheelchair user. The young girl's aspirations and her belief in her ability to achieve them could change in an instant!

For those who have a permanent disability or chronic condition, the identities portrayed by people with disability may be helpful for navigating the initial phases of disability or the experience of rehabilitation (Dunn & Burcaw, 2013). Similarly, developing a disability identity of their own can shape their views of themselves and their bodies, how they interact with the world, and their ability to adapt to their disability (Forber-Pratt et al., 2017). Recruiting and embracing students with disability for nursing education can increase the roles and opportunities of nurses.

> Nursing students with disability can model disability pride for patients and be an untapped asset for the nursing profession.

Expanding our understanding of disability from a cultural minority perspective presents a unique opportunity for nursing leadership to diversify the nursing workforce and improve culturally competent care (Marks, 2007). As with racial and ethnic minorities, including nursing students with disability in a learning environment can enhance cultural competence (Lester, 1998a, 1998b). When students without disability work alongside people with disability, the educational environment is enriched (Evans, 2005). At the same time, nursing students with disability can learn processes to promote a sense of self through mirroring, modeling, and recognition practices as they pose questions such as, "Who am I?"

Increasing nurses' understanding of the relationship between disability legislation, civil rights, disability culture and pride, and advocacy skills is critical in caring for people with disability. By reshaping and broadening disability paradigms in nursing education, nurses in clinical practice and nursing faculty can enhance the provision of culturally relevant care across all nursing specialties, cultures and populations, and settings.

ENHANCING CULTURALLY COMPETENT CARE

Increasing the supply of qualified diverse healthcare workers can enhance culturally competent care for all healthcare recipients. This includes people with disability who may—like members of other minority groups—benefit from providers who share their disability status. Culturally competent care is care that recognizes and considers people's behavior patterns, values, beliefs, and needs, and considers people's shared as well as unique experiences.

Eddey and Robey (2005) suggest that lack of cultural sensitivity or cultural competence, along with some people's tendency to avoid those with disability, may contribute to the healthcare disparities that affect the health and well-being of people with disability. Nursing students with disability can play a critical role in meeting the care needs of people with temporary and permanent disability by increasing awareness on the part of healthcare professionals without disability about the experiences of those with disability.

If nurses can model these behaviors to provide culturally competent care, it's likely other healthcare professionals will provide respectful care as well. This is because nurses serve in many leadership roles in healthcare systems. As observed by nursing leader Mary Wakefield, "Nurses find themselves at a historic juncture in the evolution of healthcare delivery, a time when they can play a pivotal leadership role" (Wakefield, 2013).

PEOPLE WITH DISABILITY DEVELOPING NEW EXPECTATIONS AND ROLES

As indicated by the improved high-school graduation rates—70% in 2015 compared to 27% in 1995—and ambitious employment goals of people with disability (Congressional Research Service, 2017), today's nursing students in the US have benefited from special education laws, beginning with the passage of the 1975 Education for All Handicapped Children Act (Public Law 94-142) and have new perspectives and expectations. In 1978—the first year *The American Freshman: National Norms* report included a question about disability status (Henderson, 1992)—the percentage of college freshmen with disability was 2.6%. Since then, it has steadily increased. In 2000, the first wave of students educated under the mandates of the Americans with Disabilities Act (ADA) of 1990 arrived on campus with new skills, expectations, and goals.

In 2010, 11.9% of incoming freshmen reported having one disability or disorder, and 2.7% said they had two or more, for a total of 14.6% (Hurtado, Pryor, Tran, DeAngelo, & Blake, 2010). In 2016, 21.9% of incoming freshmen identified having at least one disability or disorder, with 16.0% reporting one, 4.3% reporting two, and 1.6% reporting they had three or more (Eagan et al., 2017). In 2018, the *American Freshman: National Norms* report documented the following (Stolzenberg et al., 2019):

- 13.9% of students reported having a psychological disorder such as depression

- 7.4% of students reported having attention-deficit/hyperactivity disorder

- 4.6% of students reported having physical disability (e.g., speech, sight, mobility, hearing, etc.)

- 3.9% of students reported having a learning disability

- 2.8% of students reported having a chronic illness (e.g., cancer, diabetes, autoimmune disorders, etc.)

- 0.9% of students reported having autism spectrum disorder

As key contributors to the care of people with complex health conditions across the life span (Bates et al., 2018), nurses are exceptionally situated to rethink the value and roles of students and nurses with disability in nursing. As we increasingly emphasize disease and injury prevention as well as the management of health and chronic conditions, competencies in nursing—such as care coordination, health education, transitional care, and public health services—are likely to dominate care needs (O'Neil, 2009). Nurses are central in developing innovative practices and conceptualizing pioneering roles for themselves, and nurses with disability bring a fresh and distinct perspective.

CULTURALLY RELEVANT HEALTHCARE EVOLVING THROUGH ACTIVISM, ADVOCACY, AND LEGISLATION

Nurses can chart new life courses and eliminate obstacles for people with disability by sharing basic information about disability history and the ongoing successes of people with disability. In the United States, the first significant civil rights legislation pertaining to disability was the Rehabilitation Act of 1973. This legislation guaranteed access to all federally financed programs, schools, and healthcare facilities by people with disability. Under Section 504, qualified students with disability could *no longer* be excluded in postsecondary education institutions receiving federal funds.

In 1975, two organizations in the United Kingdom—the Union of the Physically Impaired Against Segregation (UPIAS) and the Disability Alliance—pushed to enable people with disability to be "more active and involved in their own affairs" (UPIAS and Disability Alliance, 1975). They argued that people with disability were not disabled by impairments but "by the disabling barriers ... faced in society" (Oliver, 2013, p. 1025).

In 1977, for the first time ever, people with disability in the United States mobilized as a community to convey the daily attitudinal and environmental barriers they encountered and to push for disability rights. They occupied US Department of Health, Education, and Welfare (HEW) buildings across the country. The longest of these sit-ins was in San Francisco, which lasted for 28 days. Their activism resulted in the issuance of regulations for Section 504. This pivotal moment acknowledged people with disability as both a community and a political force (O'Toole, 2005).

On the international front, disability activists directed their efforts toward changing the interaction between people and society regarding disability-related problems. They sought to negate the singular focus among health professionals to "cure" or "normalize" people with disability (Oliver, 1998).

Advancements achieved by the US disability community broadened our understanding of disability to include a concept called the *social model of disability*. This term emerged in 1983 and was coined by British academic, author, and disability rights activist Mike Oliver (Oliver, 2013). It describes the ideological shift that identifies societal and structural barriers as the reason people with disability are isolated and excluded from full participation in society. According to the social model of disability, being disabled is neutral; disability simply represents a difference, and societal and structural barriers limit opportunities. This stands in contrast to the medical model of disability, which suggests that being disabled is negative, disability represents a deficiency or abnormality, and that the isolation felt by people with disability is due to the disability and not to societal or structural barriers. The social model of disability is widely accepted within the international disability community. However, it, along with other models of disability that support the rights of people with disability, remains mostly absent in nursing education.

Chapter 2 discusses various models of disability in more detail.

The ADA is based on the social model of disability (Americans with Disabilities Act [ADA], 1990). However, from 1990 to 2008, the gap between the law's demands and societal attitudes prompted the courts to repeatedly narrow the statute (Burgdorf, 2005; Emens, 2012; Ragged Edge Online, 1999). Unlike other marginalized groups in the US—whose efforts to obtain civil rights were very public and sometimes bloody—Americans with disability were "empowered by civil rights legislation" *before* broad social consciousness about the circumstances and capabilities of people with disability was raised (Burke, 1997; Shapiro, 1993; Stein, 2004). So, many people without (and even with) disability lacked basic knowledge about discrimination due to disability status (Areheart, 2008). The Supreme Court and lower courts slowly barricaded the door that had been opened by the ADA by creating an overly narrow definition of "disability" and limiting who was protected by the ADA (Feldblum, 2000)— even though Congress had indicated that courts should apply the definition of disability cited in the Rehabilitation Act of 1973. Indeed, many people who had been considered disabled under the Rehabilitation Act were excluded from protection against discrimination through a variety of court decisions after the passage of the ADA (Dyer, 2011). This helps explain why employers prevailed in 91.6% of ADA legal cases during the 1990s (Joiner, 2010).

Due to this increased emphasis on determining who did and did not have a disability, more people with disability were restricted from admittance into nursing programs. Compounding this trend was a 1979 Supreme Court decision—Southeastern Community College v. Davis, 442 US 397—that allowed a nursing department at a community college in North Carolina to deny the application of a student with a hearing impairment (who, incidentally, was already a practicing licensed nurse). The court also ruled that people with disability could be required to meet technical standards, including physical qualifications (Lipton, 2017). Interestingly, with the introduction of technical standards as a result of this case, practicing nurses with disability reported anecdotally that they would have been excluded from nursing school had the technical standards been in place when they applied. Due to attitudinal and arbitrary environmental barriers within nursing schools after the passage of the ADA, becoming a nurse with disability became an unachievable dream for many students.

Technical standards are discussed in more detail in the section "Technical Standards for Education Versus Essential Functions of Employment" later in this chapter.

NURSING STUDENTS WITH DISABILITY: TRANSFORMING NURSING PRACTICE AND HEALTH OUTCOMES

According to the World Health Organization (WHO, 2011), about 15% of the global population—roughly 1 billion people—live with a disability. Many people are denied their human rights and are marginalized in their communities. Reports estimate that 80% of people with disability live in developing countries. Nurses are the largest healthcare occupational group positioned to ensure positive outcomes and to promote and protect the rights of people with disability (United Nations Department of Economic and Social Affairs, n.d.).

A classic study documented that students entering nursing programs had more positive attitudes toward people with disability than their faculty (Brillhart, Jay, & Wyers, 1990). Encouraging this innate positive attitude in our students with disability and their nondisabled peers can have a positive impact on all healthcare recipients.

Recruiting students with disability to be nurses can enhance nursing theoretical frameworks, education, practice, and research to provide culturally relevant care for everyone. However, a persistent challenge exists within the nursing profession to expand diversity—including disability—among students, practitioners, faculty, and researchers within a culturally diverse population (Institute of Medicine, 2011). Although systematic data on the types and number of disabilities among nurses are not available, data collected through the 2012 California Current Population Survey revealed that only 3% of healthcare workers are people with disability (US Census Bureau, 2012).

Developing recruitment and enrollment strategies to include students with disability supports efforts to transform healthcare by considering disability to be a difference within a limiting environment. Viewing disability as a difference allows for endless possibilities with regard to nursing care innovation (Marks, 2000), the provision of culturally congruent care, and promoting a vision that people with disability are our peers and our patients (Marks, 2007). Rethinking attitudes, instructional design, and environmental access is critical.

TECHNICAL STANDARDS FOR EDUCATION VERSUS ESSENTIAL FUNCTIONS OF EMPLOYMENT

In the late 1990s, the National Council of State Boards of Nursing (NCSBN) Nursing Practice & Education Committee released a document called "Guidelines for Using Results of Functional Abilities Studies and Other Resources" (NCSBN, 1999). The purpose of this document was to provide guidelines for the use of a series of studies initiated by the NCSBN in response to Congress' adoption of the Americans with Disabilities Act (ADA, 1990). These studies were conducted to identify competencies that nurses must possess, along with knowledge, skills, and abilities evaluated via licensing examination, to function safely and effectively in various employment settings. A section of this document, "Validation Study: Functional Abilities Essential for Nursing Practice," delineated 16 categories of functional abilities and attributes—for example, the ability to lift 25 pounds, reach below the waist, see objects 20 feet away, hear faint body sounds, and move in small spaces (Yocom, 1996).

The functional abilities were meant to be a representative list of essential skills and abilities nurses might need to possess for *employment*—not a list of skills and abilities applicants needed to be admitted into nursing school. However, many nursing programs across the country adopted the functional abilities listed in the NCSBN document as their technical standards for admission into their nursing programs (US Department of Labor Office of Disability Employment Policy, 2014). This posed a problem for students with disability because the standards often excluded them and perpetuated the impression that they represented a safety risk to themselves or others, had insurmountable health concerns, and presented programmatic or economic difficulties.

Under Section 504 of the Rehabilitation Act, schools can use technical standards, which often include a list of nonacademic skills or experiences that students must have prior to entry. Technical standards are specific to educational programs. In contrast, essential functions are applicable to specific employment settings. The essential functions of a nurse are not the same—nor should they be—as the technical standards for a nursing student. Technical standards reflect a sample of the performance abilities and characteristics that are necessary to successfully complete the requirements of a specific nursing program and are not requirements for admission into the programs (Smith, 2009; Marks & Ailey, 2014). For people with disability, an unintended outcome of the passage of the ADA relates to technical standards creating barriers to successful admission into nursing schools and essential functions for jobs being a hindrance for securing or maintaining employment.

In 2003, Rush University's College of Nursing in Chicago, Illinois hosted the first official dialogue on the subject when it convened the Symposium on Nursing Students with Disabilities. This symposium heralded a new era of diversity inclusive of people with disability in the nursing profession (Pischke-Winn, Andreoli, & Halstead, 2004). It achieved two important milestones:

- The value-added perspective of nurses with disability led to the formation of the National Organization of Nurses with Disabilities.

- It spurred an open dialogue on the impact of the "Functional Abilities Essential for Nursing Practice" document (NCSBN Nursing Practice & Education Committee, 1999) in preventing students with disability from admission into nursing academic programs.

The dialogue during the Rush symposium prompted the NCSBN to remove the "Functional Abilities Essential for Nursing Practice" document from its website. In a related development, the United Nations ratified the Convention on the Rights of Persons with Disabilities (CRPD) in 2006. Now, 30 years since the passage of the ADA and almost 15 years since the ratification of the CRPD, enrollment of students with disability in postsecondary programs continues to increase, with 14.8% of undergraduate students in health-field degree programs reporting a disability (Betz, Smith, & Bui, 2012). Still, many nursing and allied health programs across the US continue to use the NCBSN document as their technical standards for student admissions (Ailey & Marks, 2016).

Nursing schools that incorporate the social model of disability in their curricula can reframe negative stereotypes of people with disability to a value-added perspective. Moreover, faculty can reconceptualize technical standards and the fundamental requirements for nursing education. For example, rather than viewing student nurses who use a wheelchair as a safety threat—someone who might harm patients—faculty see them as having an innate understanding of useful strategies for patients with disability beyond what is taught in nursing education programs, and a natural ability to improve safety measures for patients who use wheelchairs in their homes. Or, rather than assuming a student with vision loss or blindness could be a nurse "if only he were able to see," faculty see the student as being ideally positioned to teach patients with vision loss or blindness to use various assistive devices to care for themselves, engage with their family and friends, and maintain employment.

Some nursing schools use concerns related to programmatic and economic issues to justify their rejection of students with disability. They say that changing their nursing program to accommodate these students is too difficult—an undue hardship. But adopting a universal design instruction approach can fundamentally transform nursing education for *all* students and even lead to improved patient outcomes, with minimal cost (Levey, 2018).

For more on universal design, see the sidebar "What Is Universal Design?" later in this chapter.

Many technical standards are based on skills that students will learn in the program—for example, "must be able to hear/detect a heart murmur through a stethoscope" (Smith, 2009). Because students will learn this skill in school, it is not a requirement for entering the program. Additionally, technical standards for nursing education based on the NCSBN functional abilities often focus on *how* students carry out learned skills (e.g., "must be able to talk to patients directly" or "must be able to hear a heart murmur through a stethoscope") rather than *what* the skill is meant to achieve (e.g., "must be able to communicate effectively" or "must be able to gather vital signs using a variety of means") (Smith, 2009). Developing technical standards that include a tagline, such as "able to meet these requirements with or without a reasonable accommodation," can ensure that students with disability do not experience discrimination.

Technical standards determine whether or not someone is qualified, with or without a disability. Students with disability should be afforded the opportunity to work toward meeting those standards with or without an accommodation. More contemporary technical standards allow for the admission of students who are capable of carrying out a variety of nursing tasks incorporating their disability to provide expert care across a variety of settings (Ailey & Marks, 2016; Marks & Ailey, 2014). Technical standards are written so that students with disability do not experience discrimination.

Model technical standards and objectives presented in Table 9.1 shift the focus of nursing education away from training "task-oriented" students for work in acute-care settings. Instead, the table presents nurses as knowledge workers who provide care across all types of settings. Technical standards in nursing may include the following required abilities and skills (Marks & Ailey, 2014):

- Acquiring fundamental knowledge

- Developing communication skills

- Interpreting data

- Integrating knowledge to establish clinical judgment

- Incorporating appropriate professional attitudes and behaviors into nursing practice

TABLE 9.1   TECHNICAL STANDARDS AND OBJECTIVES FOR NURSING EDUCATION PROGRAMS

REQUIREMENTS	STANDARDS	OBJECTIVES
Acquiring fundamental knowledge	Ability to learn in classroom and educational settings Ability to find sources of and acquire knowledge Ability to be a lifelong learner Novel and adaptive thinking	Acquire, conceptualize, and use evidence-based information from demonstrations and experiences in the basic and applied sciences, including but not limited to information conveyed through online coursework, lectures, group seminars, small group activities, and physical demonstrations. Develop healthcare solutions and responses beyond that which is rote or rule-based.
Developing communication skills	Communication abilities for sensitive and effective interactions with patients (persons, families, and communities) Communication abilities for effective interaction with the healthcare team (patients, their supports, other professional and nonprofessional team members) Sense-making of information gathered from communication Social intelligence	Accurately elicit and interpret information, such as medical history, to effectively evaluate a client's or patient's condition. Accurately convey information and interpretation of information using one or more means of communication—verbal, written, assisted (such as TTY) or electronic—to patients and the healthcare team. Effectively communicate within teams. Determine a deeper meaning or significance in what is being expressed. Connect with others to sense and stimulate reactions and desired interactions.
Interpreting data	Ability to observe patient conditions and responses to health and illness Ability to assess and monitor health needs Computational thinking Cognitive load management	Obtain and interpret information from assessment maneuvers, such as assessing respiratory and cardiac function, blood pressure, blood sugar, and neurological status.

continues

TABLE 9.1 TECHNICAL STANDARDS AND OBJECTIVES FOR NURSING EDUCATION PROGRAMS (CONT.)

REQUIREMENTS	STANDARDS	OBJECTIVES
Interpreting data (cont.)		Obtain and interpret information from diagnostic representations of physiologic phenomena during a comprehensive assessment of patients.
		Obtain and interpret information from assessment of a patient's environment and responses to health across the continuum.
		Obtain and interpret for evaluation information about responses to nursing action.
		Translate data into abstract concepts and to understand data-based reasoning.
Integrating knowledge to establish clinical judgment	Critical thinking, problem-solving, and decision-making abilities to care for persons, families, or communities across the health continuum and within (or managing or improving) their environments, in one or more environments of care	Accomplish, direct, or interpret assessment of persons, families, or communities; develop, implement, and evaluate plans of care; or direct the development, implementation, and evaluation of care.
	Intellectual and conceptual abilities to accomplish the essentials of the nursing program (for example, baccalaureate essentials)	Critically assess and develop content that uses new media forms and leverage these media for persuasive communication.
	New-media literacy	Have literacy in and an ability to understand concepts across disciplines.
	Transdisciplinarity	Represent and develop tasks
	Design mindset	and work processes for desired outcomes.

Incorporating appropriate professional attitudes and behaviors into nursing practice	Concern for others, integrity, ethical conduct, account-ability, interest, and motiva-tion	Maintain effective, mature, and sensitive relationships with clients/patients, students, faculty, staff, and other profes-sionals in all circumstances.
	Interpersonal skills for professional interactions with a diverse population of individuals, families, and communities	Make proper judgments re-garding safe and quality care.
		Function effectively under stress and adapt to changing environments inherent in clini-cal practice.
	Interpersonal skills for pro-fessional interactions with members of the healthcare team, including patients, their supports, other health-care professionals, and team members	Demonstrate professional role in interactions with patients and intra- and interprofes-sional teams.
	Skills for promoting change for necessary quality health-care	Operate in different cultural settings (including disability culture).
	Cross-cultural competency	Work productively, drive en-gagement, and demonstrate presence as a member of a virtual team.
	Virtual collaboration	

Innovative technical standards for nursing education can also incorporate a set of competencies outlined in a document called "Essentials for Baccalaureate Education" put forth by the American Association of Colleges of Nursing (AACN). This document includes coverage of areas such as the following (AACN, 2008; Marks & Ailey, 2014):

- Patient-centered care
- Interprofessional teams
- Evidence-based practice
- Quality improvement
- Patient safety
- Informatics
- Clinical reasoning/critical thinking

- Genetics and genomics
- Cultural sensitivity
- Professionalism
- Practice across the lifespan
- End-of-life care

A RENEWED ERA OF EQUALITY THROUGH THE ADA AMENDMENT ACT

Multiple legal court decisions—many of which focused on the definitional bounds of disability (essentially, the medical model of disability) rather than on discrimination (at the core of the social model of disability)—resulted in the loss of many ADA safeguards (Areheart, 2008). In response to several Supreme Court decisions that narrowly interpreted the ADA definition of disability, the US Congress passed the Americans with Disabilities Act Amendments Act (ADAAA) of 2008 (ADA Amendments Act of 2008). The ADAAA, which became effective on January 1, 2009, aimed to reinforce protections from discrimination based on disability using the social model of disability (Dyer, 2011) and reaffirmed President George H. W. Bush's assertion that "every man, woman, and child with a disability can now pass through once-closed doors into a bright new era of equality, independence, and freedom" (Bush, 1990). President George W. Bush rekindled the spirit of the ADA by addressing the ongoing attitudinal barriers that impeded people with disability and implementing the ADA's original objectives by "reinstating a broad scope of protection to be available under the ADA" (Hensel, 2009, p. 2).

The ADAAA significantly expanded the ADA's definition of disability to ensure even broader coverage for people with disability. It clarified that an "impairment" that is "episodic or in remission" is a disability if, when it is active, it substantially limits a major life activity (Dyer, 2011), and stated that disability status relates to the disability in its unmitigated state (e.g., without the effect of aids such as eyeglasses, medication, or prosthetics) (Dyer, 2011). Finally, it shifted the focus from "does an individual have a disability?" to "were efforts made to accommodate that person?"

Today, with the ADAAA's clarification of the definition of disability, students and employees are increasingly requesting—and receiving—accommodations (Husband & Williams, 2010). Under the ADAAA, the failure of nursing schools to provide appropriate accommodations to nursing students is potentially discriminatory (Job Accommodation Network [JAN], 2011). By attending to the interactive process of providing accommodations, organizations—including nursing schools—can minimize their exposure to compensatory and punitive damages (Husband & Williams, 2010).

> Operationalizing ADAAA protections provides an opportunity for nurse educators and administrators to rethink the "what" of nursing practice; how nurses with disability can expand nursing knowledge, skills, and abilities; and how nurses with disability can promote safe and culturally competent nursing care.

INCREASED EMPLOYMENT AND SECTION 503 OF THE REHABILITATION ACT OF 1973

Despite federal legislation supporting the rights of people with disability, people with disability continue to struggle to obtain nursing education and employment in healthcare. Moreover, educational programs across all areas of healthcare still lack proactive discussion regarding the inherent value of people with disability as healthcare professionals.

As part of a continuing effort to strengthen the enforcement of the ADA and the ADAAA, the US government revised regulations in Section 503 of the Rehabilitation Act of 1973. These new regulations, which are enforced by the US Office of Federal Contract =Compliance Programs, pertain to the recruitment, hiring, promotion, and retention of people with disability by employers with federal contracts. Specifically, they require these employers to ensure that 7% of their workforce consists of qualified people with disability in each of their job groups, including healthcare, and report their progress in achieving this goal. This represents the first single national utilization goal for people with disability (ADA National Network, 2014). Nursing faculty have a critical role in promoting the 7% rule in clinical sites and educational programs (e.g., hiring faculty with disability).

SEEING NURSES WITH DISABILITY AS OUR PEERS

According to the "2007–2008 California Survey of People with Disabilities" report, 97% of unemployed survey respondents said they were not working because a healthcare provider had told them they couldn't work (Kaye, 2010). This may help explain why about 21% of people with disability in the US are employed, compared to 69% of people without disability.

By increasing the number of healthcare professionals with disability, we can promote social change for people with disability and address the persistent underrepresentation of people with disability in the US healthcare workforce. Nurses with disability often innovate new clinical skills and practices that can create new employment possibilities, improve the healthcare system, and demonstrate for people with disability that they can work. With the support of changes to Section 503 of the Rehabilitation Act, nurses have a pivotal role in altering our perceptions of the value of people with disability in healthcare and support civil rights for students and nurses with disability.

NURSE SHORTAGES AND NURSES WITH DISABILITY CREATE WORKFORCE INNOVATION

The US Bureau of Labor Statistics indicates that the number of registered nurse positions in the US is expected to grow from 2.9 million in 2016 to 3.4 million in 2026—an increase of 15%. This includes more than 200,000 new registered nurses each year to fill newly created nursing positions and to replace nurses who are retiring (US Bureau of Labor Statistics, 2017). Additionally, experts predict a shortage of nurse practitioners in the years to come. These shortages present an opportunity to encourage and recruit people with disability to consider a career as a nurse or nurse practitioner.

Understanding disability rights activism and legislation supports efforts to expand nursing practice and to consider the variety of ways in which nursing skills can be performed. For example, some hospitals systems have begun using text messaging rather than telephones to communicate. This is useful for practitioners and patients who are Deaf or hard of hearing. Text-based messaging is also a great way to prevent communication errors and to systematically document communication by healthcare professionals.

Integrating technology into practice and including more practitioners with disability may prove invaluable in using principles of universal design and teaching these principles to patients with different abilities and learning styles. Studies have shown that incorporating universal design in clinical environments (and universal design instruction in educational experiences) can support positive self-image and health outcomes for people with disability and chronic health conditions (Marks & Ailey, 2014). As nurses with disability develop innovative approaches to nursing practice that incorporate technology, universal design, and universal design instruction, exciting new roles for people with disability and chronic conditions may emerge.

WHAT IS UNIVERSAL DESIGN?

The aim of universal design (UD) is for products, environments, and communication strategies to be usable by as many people as possible, regardless of age, ability, or situation (US Department of Labor Office of Disability Employment Policy, 2020). This concept is also referred to as inclusive design, design-for-all, lifespan design, barrier-free design, and human-centered design.

UD is a design approach based in the belief that the broad range of human ability is ordinary, not special. As such, UD accommodates people with disability, older adults, children, and others in a way that is not stigmatizing and benefits all users. The underlying premise of UD is that if it works well for people across the spectrum of functional ability, it will work better for everyone.

The following are examples of UD in action:

- Developing medication labels that can be read by people with low vision makes them easier for everyone to read.
- Minimizing external noises for classroom setting makes it easier for everyone to hear.
- Building entrances without stairs is useful for people who are pushing strollers, carrying groceries, or using a wheelchair.

Products, environments, and communication strategies (including universal design instruction) can be made usable for all people by incorporating designs that include the five senses: sight, touch, smell, taste, and hearing. Keeping a broad range of users in mind from the beginning of the design process can increase usability without significantly increasing cost.

NEW NURSING COMPETENCIES AND DIVERSE "WAYS OF KNOWING"

According to the 2011 Institute of Medicine (IOM) Report, nurses are developing new competencies in the following areas:

- Bridging the healthcare access and coverage gap
- Coordinating complex care for a diverse group of healthcare recipients
- Fulfilling the role of primary care provider
- Implementing systemwide changes to connect nursing care to safety and quality of care
- Documenting the economic value of nursing practice

Nursing students and nurses with disability bring a distinct set of skills and "ways of knowing" that can advance healthcare and help deliver culturally relevant care to all healthcare recipients (Marks & Ailey, 2014). For example, patients with disability and their families may find that nurses with

Nurses with disability represent a diverse group with unique skills to transform "ways of knowing" in healthcare education, research, and practice (Marks & Ailey, 2014).

disability enhance communication and linguistic congruency (Evans & Marks, 2009). Their shared experiences may result in greater patient involvement with healthcare, improved patient satisfaction, and enhanced health outcomes (Marks, 2007).

Nurses with disability can also develop new and innovative practices that eliminate access gaps based on their own disability experiences. An example might be a nurse who uses a wheelchair in a community nursing practice providing health-promotion and disease-prevention services to people with spinal-cord injuries. Another example could be a nurse with one hand providing care for patients who have had a hand amputation or have experienced reduced hand function. A nurse with one hand may have a unique capacity to teach patients how to use one-handed self-care strategies and develop novel practices to improve standards of care for *all* healthcare recipients.

Similar to the way racial and ethnic diversity among healthcare providers improves the quality of healthcare (Betancourt, Green, & Carrillo, 2002; Cooper-Patrick et al., 1999; Morales, Cunningham, Brown, Liu, & Hays, 1999; Saha, Arbelaez, & Cooper, 2003; Saha, Komaromy, Koepsell, & Bindman, 1999; Saha, Taggart, Komaromy, & Bindman, 2000), students and nurses with disability who bring their diverse experiences to their practice can potentially improve healthcare access and quality (Marks, 2007). Recruiting students and nurses with different life experiences can help ensure safety and quality of care as well as enable healthcare providers to coordinate care for a wide range of patients within their communities. For example, patients with and without disability often request healthcare providers who are Deaf or hard of hearing because they are more "active listeners" (R. M. Toscano, personal communication, June 11, 2013).

On a related note, although nurses who are Deaf or hard of hearing are often assumed to be a safety liability (no data support this perception) (Institute of Medicine Committee on Quality of Health Care in America, 2000), they may actually enhance patient safety and care. For example, nurses who are Deaf or hard of hearing

---

and proficient in American Sign Language (ASL) or lip-reading can improve direct communication and the provision of safe care among people who rely on these methods of communication. Additionally, not having to rely on an interpreter is likely useful and appreciated by people who are Deaf or hard of hearing while receiving psychotherapy or making life-altering healthcare decisions.

> Disability legislation and activism have energized a new generation of people with disability and chronic conditions—including healthcare professionals. Indeed, the impact that health professionals with disability can have on health outcomes for all healthcare recipients can be clearly seen.

Finally, nurses with disability report being hyper-vigilant, as they have experienced the impact of unsafe nursing care (National Organization of Nurses with Disabilities, personal communication, August 15, 2015). This may improve the care they provide.

ACCOMMODATIONS FOR PEOPLE WITH DISABILITY

Accommodations for people with disability can be beneficial in changing practice and enhancing care for patients. However, these are sometimes met with resistance, due to the assumption that unlike traditional civil rights remedies, disability accommodations are costly. However, this assumption is not factually correct. According to Stein (2004), changing the prejudicial status quo for *all* civil rights actions—including actions for equality related to gender, race, ethnicity, and sexual orientation—has associated costs. Stein (2004) states that accommodation costs for disability are similar to expenses related to ameliorating discrimination on the basis of sex or race.

In addition to remedying historical exclusion, research shows that workplace accommodations for people with disability are low cost *and* improve the workplace in many ways (JAN, 2020). According to JAN's (2020) ongoing survey of employers about workplace accommodations since 2004 across a broad range of industry sectors and sizes, benefits of workplace accommodations include the following:

- Retention of valuable employees

- Improved productivity and morale

- Reduction in workers' compensation and training costs

- Enhanced company diversity

JAN survey results also show that 58% of accommodations cost US $0, and other accommodations typically cost US $500. The cost of many of these accommodations can be shared through state-based vocational rehabilitation services (JAN, 2018).

> Some postsecondary universities have achieved compliance with necessary accommodations by offering extra credit to health professional students who assist students with disability—for example, by taking notes for them in class (Marks & Ailey, 2014).

USING THE EDUCATE FRAMEWORK TO EXPAND DIVERSITY

Nurse educators and administrators have a pivotal role in expanding diversity in nursing and increasing understanding of disability culture and disability discrimination in order to:

- Accept students and nurses with disability as valued professionals within the healthcare multidisciplinary team

- Provide culturally relevant healthcare that is accessible to all

The EDUCATE acronym serves as a framework for strategic planning to recruit and retain students and nurses with disability (Marks & Ailey, 2014). This framework aims to build capacity among faculty, administrators, students, clinical preceptors, and disability services for professionals. The acronym stands for:

- **Encourage:** Encourage conversation between faculty, clinical sites, and disability student services about the use of technical standards and the potential for discrimination that may preclude admission for students with disability (Helms, Jorgensen, & Andersen, 2006).

- **Disseminate:** Disseminate information about and examples of developing accommodations to facilitate knowledge and self-efficacy among faculty and clinical sites. Create collaborative partnerships with clinical practicum sites to increase accessibility.

- **Understand:** Understand the unique role of technical standards for education and essential functions for employment. Develop clear guidelines for recruiting, retaining, and promoting students and nurses with disability.

- **Create:** Create training hubs for advocacy skills, adaptive technology, and disability resources within nursing programs for the benefit of all students—not just those with disability—so that students and faculty will be able to provide these resources to patients.

- **Adopt:** Adopt technical standards and policies that are uniformly applied to guide advocacy for and support of students with disability in admission, matriculation, and graduation. Adhering to rigid technical standards promotes inconsistencies across students.

- **Train:** Train faculty, students, clinical sites, and disability student services on strategies to integrate disability history, civil rights legislation, and the social model of disability into existing curricula. This information is critical for people with disability and their supports. Many people with disability do not have family or friends who share their disability status. Understanding disability culture is critical for people with disability to live, learn, work, and play in their communities.

- **Ensure:** Ensure data collection is undertaken related to the participation and successes of students with disability.

Following are several resources to assist you with each aspect of the EDUCATE framework.

ENCOURAGE

- **Association on Higher Education And Disability (AHEAD) (https://www.ahead.org/home):** AHEAD addresses current and emerging issues related to disability, education, and accessibility to achieve universal access and facilities and facilitate discussion between faculty and disability student services to ensure full, effective participation by individuals with disabilities.

- **Alliance for Disability in Health Care Education (http://www.adhce.org):** ADHCE works to integrate disability-related content and experiences into healthcare education and offers training programs for medical school faculty, nursing school faculty, and other healthcare educators.

- **Office of Student Disability Services:** Students with disability should work with their school's Office of Student Disability Services to document their disability and request accommodation(s) as needed for instructional activities, facilities, programs, or services. Faculty should collaborate with Disability Services for ongoing training, in-services, and continuing education related to issues such as accommodations, legal issues, rights, and responsibilities.

DISSEMINATE

- Coalition for Disability Access in Health Science Education (https://www.hsmcoalition.org): This coalition supports the development and dissemination of best practices for facilitating access within graduate professional health science programs.

- State Boards of Nursing (BON): Faculty should know what their state's BON says about students with disability and required accommodations. They should also work with their BON to develop inclusive regulations for nurses with disability.

UNDERSTAND

- National Organization of Nurses with Disabilities (NOND) (https://nond.org): NOND promotes best practices in education and employment by providing information to individuals, nursing and disability organizations, and educational and healthcare institutions.

- "Technical Standards for Nursing Education Programs in the 21st Century" by S. H. Ailey and B. Marks (https://www.ncbi.nlm.nih.gov/pubmed/27197703): This 2017 journal article in *Rehabilitation Nursing* presents a new model of technical standards for nursing education to foster a diverse set of skills and talent.

CREATE

- ADA National Network (https://adata.org): ADA National Network provides information, guidance, and training on the Americans with Disabilities Act (ADA). It can tailor information to meet the needs of education, business, government, and people at local, regional, and national levels.

- The Association of Medical Professionals with Hearing Losses (AMPHL) (https://www.amphl.org): The AMPHL promotes advocacy and mentorship, along with the development of products (such as see-through surgical masks) to assist medical professionals (and patients) with hearing loss.

- The JAN Workplace Accommodation Toolkit (https://askjan.org/toolkit/The-JAN-Workplace-Accommodation-Toolkit.cfm): This is a free, comprehensive online resource for employers who seek to move beyond basic compliance with the ADA to create a more disability-inclusive workplace.

ADOPT

- American Association of Colleges of Nursing (AACN): Accommodating Students with Disabilities (https://www.aacnnursing.org/Education-Resources/Tool-Kits/Accommodating-Students-with-Disabilities): This web page offers resources related to technical standards for schools of nursing, such as the 2014 "White Paper on Inclusion of Students with Disabilities in Nursing Educational Programs" by B. Marks and S. Ailey.

- Open the Door, Get 'Em a Locker: Educating Nursing Students with Disabilities (https://www.youtube.com/watch?v=q3WQtR7yUpI): This is a documentary film about a nursing student with disability who used a wheelchair in nursing school and later worked as a licensed registered nurse. Educators can use this film (and its corresponding booklet) to facilitate an in-depth discussion on how to accept and promote students with a variety of disabilities in classroom and clinical settings.

TRAIN

- **Disability Studies Quarterly: Schools with Disability Studies Degrees (http://dsq-sds.org/article/view/963/1147):** This page offers a list of disability studies programs around the world. These programs are good collaborative partners for nursing students.

- **Disability History Museum (DHM) (http://www. disabilitymuseum.org):** DHM is a virtual project rather than a bricks-and-mortar museum. It aims to provide people with and without disability—including researchers, teachers, and students—a wide array of information and tools to deepen their understanding of human variation and difference and to expand their appreciation of how vital the experiences of people with disability have always been to all of our lives. The museum's digital exhibits aim to change cultural values, explore notions of identity, and discover laws and policies that have shaped the experiences of people with disability, their families, and their communities over time.

- **University of Illinois at Chicago: Bodies of Work (https:// ahs.uic.edu/disability-human-development/community- partners/bodies-of-work):** This project uses art to illuminate the experience and advance the rights of people with disability. Art showcases and celebrates the disability experience of people who have unique bodies and minds to widen society's understanding of what it means to be human.

ENSURE

- **Rush University (http://www.rushu.rush.edu):** Rush University has been at the forefront of healthcare institutions promoting disability rights, the ADA, and Section 504 of the Rehabilitation Act of 1973. The Rush ADA Task Force oversees its ADA transition plan to develop "programs related to disability rights and accommodations" that make its university and medical center more accessible for improved access and services, outreach, and education (Rush University, n.d.). The Rush ADA Task Force also develops questionnaires that capture the qualitative and quantitative success of students and nurses with disability, along with their impact on patients, peers, faculty, and employers.

Students and nurses with disability live in societies that routinely devalue disability despite legislative mandates. Additionally, many students with disability who are just beginning their nursing education may not have had an opportunity to learn and articulate the value of their own experiences as people with disability. The same is true of nurses who acquire disability later in their career.

An exciting opportunity exists to transform nursing education and practice. Supporting students and nurses with disability and identifying effective accommodation and universal design strategies can open more nursing employment opportunities, enhance healthcare services, strengthen the nursing workforce, and improve health outcomes for all healthcare recipients.

THE NEED FOR SYSTEM-WIDE CHANGE IN NURSING EDUCATION

Nurses constitute the largest part of the professional health workforce. All around the world, nurses are often the first—and sometimes the only—health professionals that people see. The quality of their initial assessment, care, and treatment is vital. Nurses must be able to use their knowledge and skills to the fullest (All-Party Parliamentary Group on Global Health, 2016).

Unfortunately, healthcare professionals, including nurses, often unwittingly display prejudicial behavior around people with disability. This perpetuates a medical-model view that relies on unfounded stereotypical assumptions that people with disability are "less than" people without. These attitudinal biases can negatively affect quality of care, including *diagnostic overshadowing*, in which a person's symptoms are attributed to their disability rather than an emerging health condition (Javaid, Nakata, & Michael 2019; Lewis & Stenfert-Krese, 2010). They also explain why some people with disability state that they are often treated as a diagnosis rather than as a human being. This creates an unnecessary obstacle to providing quality care for this population. Along with these attitudinal barriers, people with disability face other barriers, such as inaccessible healthcare buildings, facilities, and equipment.

Expanding nursing curricula to include coverage of the history of disability, legislation pertaining to disability, and the culture and capabilities of people with disability can have an enormous impact on the provision of care for all healthcare recipients. At present, few healthcare professions' educational programs adequately address disability issues in their curricula, if they address them at all (Havercamp & Scott, 2015; Holder, Waldman, & Hood, 2009; Minihan et al., 2004; Thierer & Meyerowitz, 2005). Adhering solely to a medicalized view of people with disability perpetuates the attitude that students with disability will be unable to work as a nurse due to their perceived "impairments."

The need to improve nursing curricula to include disability education becomes even more clear when one considers the results of a 1990 study by Brillhart and colleagues, which compared the attitudes of nursing students, nursing educators, various nursing professionals, and people with disability toward people with disability (Brillhart et al., 1990). Not surprisingly people with disability demonstrated the most positive attitudes toward this population. However, the attitudes of nursing students, nursing graduate students, and nursing educators were progressively less positive, in that order. This suggests that nursing students receive these negative attitudes from faculty during their nursing education.

By incorporating the intent and spirit of legislation (such as the ADAAA and Section 503 of the Rehabilitation Act of 1973) and disability activism into curricula, we can begin to dismantle environmental barriers and address cultural attitudes, biases, and social behaviors. Ensuring disability-friendly regulations, policies, procedures, and practices can support people with disability to enter and stay in the nursing profession (Marks & Ailey, 2014) and can improve the delivery of high-quality care.

Health professionals with disability who have a strong sense of disability identity and pride can model a positive image for their colleagues and healthcare recipients and help remove attitudinal barriers. Students and nurses with disability and chronic conditions can be assets to the nursing profession *because* of their disability experiences and insights. Embracing our nursing colleagues with disability creates a unique niche for modeling disability pride, which can enhance care and change lives. We can focus on developing strategies that facilitate the success of people with disability in nursing education and nursing practice and stop questioning whether people with disability can be nurses (Marks, 2007).

SUMMARY

This chapter addressed the need for systematic capacity-building in nursing education to recruit and retain nurses with disability as peers in the nursing workforce. The ethical and professional mandates to do so were addressed, along with a discussion of legislation that requires their inclusion in nursing education. With their unique perspectives, nurses with disability can increase the diversity of the nursing workforce; enhance the knowledge, skill, and attitudes of nurses across healthcare settings; and improve healthcare and health outcomes of people with disability.

The EDUCATE framework discussed in this chapter, along with the specific examples and suggestions, can be incorporated into strategic planning to recruit and retain students and nurses with disability and expand diversity in nursing. Understanding disability from a multicultural perspective can redefine clinical skills through new "ways of knowing" that become standard practice. Nurses can promote equity for people with disability and healthcare access.

REFERENCES

ADA Amendments Act of 2008, Pub. L. No.110-325, 122 Stat. 3553 (2008).

ADA National Network. (2014). Section 503 of the Rehabilitation Act rules. Retrieved from https://adata.org/factsheet/section-503

Ailey, S. H., & Marks, B. (2016). Technical standards for nursing education programs in the 21st century. *Rehabilitation Nursing*. doi:10.1002/rnj.278

All-Party Parliamentary Group on Global Health. (2016). Triple impact: How developing nursing will improve health, promote gender equality and support economic growth. *World Health Organization*. Retrieved from https://www.who.int/hrh/com-heeg/digital-APPG_triple-impact.pdf?ua=1&ua=1

American Association of Colleges of Nursing. (2008). The essentials of baccalaureate education for professional nursing practice. Retrieved from https://www.aacnnursing.org/Portals/42/Publications/BaccEssentials08.pdf

American Nurses Association. (2020). Nursing workforce development. Retrieved from https://ana.aristotle.com/SitePages/nursingworkforcedevelopment.aspx

Americans with Disabilities Act of 1990, 42 U.S.C. § 12101 (1990).

Areheart, B. A. (2008). When disability isn't "just right": The entrenchment of the medical model of disability and the Goldilocks dilemma. *Indiana Law Journal, 83*(1), 181–232.

Bates, R. A., Blair, L. M., Schlegel, E. C., McGovern, C. M., Nist, M. D., Sealschott, S., & Arcoleo, K. (2018). Nursing across the lifespan: Implications of lifecourse theory for nursing research. *Journal of Pediatric Health Care, 32*(1), 92–97. doi:10.1016/j.pedhc.2017.07.006

Betancourt, J. R., Green, A. R., & Carrillo, J. E. (2002). Cultural competence in health care: Emerging frameworks and practical approaches. *The Commonwealth Fund.* Retrieved from https://www.commonwealthfund.org/sites/default/files/documents/___media_files_publications_fund_report_2002_oct_cultural_competence_in_health_care__emerging_frameworks_and_practical_approaches_betancourt_culturalcompetence_576_pdf.pdf

Betz, C. L., Smith, K., & Bui, K. (2012). A survey of California nursing programs: Admission and accommodation policies for students with disabilities. *Journal of Nursing Education, 51*(12), 676. doi: 10.3928/01484834-20121112-01

Bogart, K. (2020). How disability pride fights ableism: Reflections on the 30th anniversary of the Americans with Disabilities Act. *Psychology Today.* Retrieved from https://www.psychologytoday.com/us/blog/disability-is-diversity/202008/how-disability-pride-fights-ableism

Brillhart, B. A., Jay, H., & Wyers, M. E. (1990). Attitudes toward people with disabilities. *Rehabilitation Nursing, 15*(2), 80–85. doi:10.1002/j.2048-7940.1990.tb01439.x

Burgdorf, R. L. (2005). *Some lessons on equality from the Americans with Disabilities Act.* [White Paper.] Cardiff, UK: Cardiff University.

Burke, T. (1997). The Americans with Disabilities Act: On the rights track. In P. Nivola (Ed.), *Comparative disadvantage? Domestic social regulations and the global economy* (pp. 242–318). Washington D.C.: The Brookings Institution.

Bush, G. W. (1990). Remarks of President George H. W. Bush at the signing of the Americans with Disabilities Act. Retrieved from http://www.ada.gov/ghw_bush_ada_remarks.html

Congressional Research Service. (2017). Students with disabilities graduating from high school and entering postsecondary education: In brief. Retrieved from https://www.everycrsreport.com/reports/R44887.html

Cooper-Patrick, L., Gallo, J. J., Gonzales, J. J., Vu, H. T., Powe, N. R., Nelson, C., & Ford, D. E. (1999). Race, gender, and partnership in the patient-physician relationship. *JAMA, 282*(6), 583–589.

Dunn, D. S., & Burcaw, S. (2013). Thinking about disability identity: Major themes of disability are explored. *Spotlight on Disability Newsletter.* Retrieved from https://www.apa.org/pi/disability/resources/publications/newsletter/2013/11/disability-identity

Dyer, S. (May, 2011). An overview of ADAAA and other disability legislation compliance issues: A white paper. Oklahoma City, OK: Association on Higher Education and Disability.

Eagan, K., Stolzenberg, E. B., Zimmerman, H. B., Aragon, M. C., Sayson, H. W., & Rios-Aguilar, C. (2017). The American freshman: National norms fall 2016. *University of California Los Angeles (UCLA) Higher Education Research Institute (HERI).* Retrieved from https://www.heri.ucla.edu/monographs/TheAmericanFreshman2016.pdf

Eddey, G. E., & Robey, K. L. (2005). Considering the culture of disability in cultural competence education. *Academic Medicine, 80*(7), 706–712. doi:10.1097/00001888-200507000-00019

Emens, E. F. (2012). Disabling attitudes: U.S. disability law and the ADA Amendments Act. *The American Journal of Comparative Law, 60*(1), 205–234. doi:10.5131/AJCL.2011.0020

Evans, B. (2005). Nursing education for students with disabilities: Our students, our teachers. In M. Oermann, & K. Heinrich (Eds.), *Strategies for Teaching, Assessment, and Program Planning* (pp. 3-22). (*Annual Review of Nursing Education;* Vol. 3).

Evans, B., & Marks, B. A. (2009). Open the door, get 'em a locker: Educating nursing students with disabilities. Retrieved from https://www.youtube.com/watch?v=q3WQtR7yUpI

Feldblum, C. R. (2000). Definition of disability under federal anti-discrimination law: What happened? Why? And what can we do about it? *Berkeley Journal of Employment and Labor Law, 21,* 91.

Forber-Pratt, A. J., Lyew, D. A., Mueller, C., & Samples, L. B. (2017). Disability identity development: A systematic review of the literature. *Rehabilitation Psychology, 62*(2), 198–207. doi:10.1037/rep0000134

Havercamp, S. M., & Scott, H. M. (2015). National health surveillance of adults with disabilities, adults with intellectual and developmental disabilities, and adults with no disabilities. *Disability & Health Journal, 8*(2), 165–172. doi:10.1016/j.dhjo.2014.11.002

Helms, L., Jorgensen, J., & Andersen, M. A. (2006). Disability law and nursing education: An update. *Journal of Professional Nursing, 22*(3), 190-6. doi:10.1016/j.profnurs.2006.03.005

Henderson, C. (1992). College freshman with disabilities: A statistical profile. Retrieved from https://files.eric.ed.gov/fulltext/ED354792.pdf

Hensel, W. F. (2009). Rights resurgence: The impact of the ADA Amendments Act on schools and universities. *Georgia State University Law Review*. Retrieved from https://ssrn.com/abstract=1393776

Holder, M., Waldman, H. B., & Hood, H. (2009). Preparing health professionals to provide care to individuals with disabilities. *International Journal of Oral Science, 1*(2), 66–71. doi:10.4248/ijos.09022

Hurtado, S., Pryor, J. H., Tran, S., DeAngelo, L., & Blake, L. P. (2010). The American freshman: National norms fall 2010. *University of California Los Angeles (UCLA) Higher Education Research Institute (HERI)*. Retrieved from https://heri.ucla.edu/PDFs/pubs/briefs/HERI_ResearchBrief_Norms2010.pdf

Husband, J. M., & Williams, B. J. (2010). You just might find...you get what you need—A practical guide to finding and managing disability accommodations. *Holland & Hart*. Retrieved from https://www.hollandhart.com/articles/YouJustMightFindYouGetWhatYouNeed.pdf

Iezzoni, L. I. (2016). Why increasing numbers of physicians with disability could improve care for patients with disability. *AMA Journal of Ethics, 18*(10), 1,041–1,049. doi:10.1001/journalofethics.2016.18.10.msoc2-1610

Institute of Education Sciences National Center for Education Statistics. (2019). Digest of education statistics 2017. Retrieved from https://files.eric.ed.gov/fulltext/ED592104.pdf

Institute of Medicine. (2011). *The future of nursing: Leading change, advancing health*. Washington, DC: National Academies Press.

Institute of Medicine Committee on Quality of Health Care in America. (2000). *To err is human: Building a safer health system*. Washington, DC: National Academies Press.

Javaid, A., Nakata, V., & Michael, D. (2019). Diagnostic overshadowing in learning disability: Think beyond the disability. *Progress in Neurology and Psychiatry, 23*(2), 8–10. doi:10.1002/pnp.531

Job Accommodation Network. (2011). Accommodation and compliance series: The ADA Amendments Act of 2008. *US Fish & Wildlife Service*. Retrieved from https://www.fws.gov/pacific/aba/dcr/training/Reasonable%20Accommodations/Handout%20-%20JAN_ADAAA.pdf

Job Accommodation Network. (2018). Spotlight series: Funding resources. Retrieved from https://askjan.org/publications/Topic-Downloads.cfm?pubid=381875

Job Accommodation Network. (2020). Benefits and costs of accommodation. Retrieved from https://askjan.org/topics/costs.cfm?csSearch=2528096_1

Joiner, A. M. (2010). The ADAAA: Opening the floodgates. *San Diego Law Review, 47*(2), 331–369.

Kaye, H. S. (2010). Barriers to employment for people with disabilities: Bad advice, poor health, and ineffective public policy. *Disability & Health Journal, 3*(2), e6. doi:10.1016/j.dhjo.2009.08.087

Lester, N. (1998a). Cultural competence: A nursing dialogue. *American Journal of Nursing, 98*(8), 26–33.

Lester, N. (1998b). Cultural competence: A nursing dialogue part 2. *American Journal of Nursing, 98*(9), 36–42.

Lewis, S., & Stenfert-Kroese, B. (2010). An investigation of nursing staff attitudes and emotional reactions towards patients with intellectual disability in a general hospital setting. *Journal of Applied Research in Intellectual Disabilities, 23*(4), 355–365. doi: 10.1111/j.1468-3148.2009.00542.x

Levey, J. A. (2018). Universal design for instruction in nursing education: An integrative review. *Nursing Education Perspectives, 39*(3), 156–161. 10.1097/01. NEP.0000000000000249

Marks, B. A. (2000). Jumping through hoops and walking on egg shells or discrimination, hazing, and abuse of students with disabilities? *Journal of Nursing Education, 39*(5), 205–210.

Marks, B. (2007). Cultural competence revisited: Nursing students with disabilities. *Journal of Nursing Education, 46*(2), 70–74. doi:10.3928/01484834-20070201-06

Marks, B., & Ailey, S. A. (2014). White paper on inclusion of students with disabilities in nursing educational programs for the California Committee on Employment of People with Disabilities (CCEPD). *American Association of Colleges of Nursing.* Retrieved from https://www.aacnnursing.org/Portals/42/AcademicNursing/Tool%20Kits/Student-Disabilities-White-Paper.pdf

Minihan, P. M., Bradshaw, Y. S., Long-Bellil, L. M., Altman, W., Perduta-Fulginiti, S., Ector, J., ... Sneiron, R. (2004). Teaching about disability: Involving patients with disabilities as medical educators. *Disability Studies Quarterly, 24*(4). doi:10.18061/ dsq.v24i4.883

Morales, L. S., Cunningham, W. E., Brown, J. A., Liu, H., & Hays, R. D. (1999). Are Latinos less satisfied with communication by health care providers? *Journal of General Internal Medicine, 14*(7), 409–417. doi:10.1046/j.1525-1497.1999.06198.x

National Council of State Boards of Nursing Nursing Practice & Education Committee. (1999). *Guidelines for using results of functional abilities studies and other resources.* Chicago, IL: National Council of State Boards of Nursing.

National Council on Disability. (2003). People with disabilities and postsecondary education—Position paper. Retrieved from https://ncd.gov/publications/2003/people-disabilities-and-postsecondary-education-position-paper

Oliver, M. (1998). Theories of disability in health practice and research. *BMJ, 317*(7170), 1,446–1,449. doi:10.1136/bmj.317.7170.1446

Oliver, M. (2013). The social model of disability: Thirty years on. *Disability & Society, 28*(7), 1,024–1,026. doi:10.1080/09687599.2013.818773

O'Neil, E. (2009). Four factors that guarantee health care change. *Journal of Professional Nursing, 25*(6), 317–321. doi:10.1016/j.profnurs.2009.10.004

O'Toole, C. J. (2005). Early days in Berkeley, and where we are now. *Ragged Edge Online.* Retrieved from http://www.raggededgemagazine.com/departments/ reflections/000499.html

Pischke-Winn, K. A., Andreoli, K. G., & Halstead, L. K. (2004). Students with disabilities: Nursing education and practice proceedings manual. *National Council of State Boards of Nursing.* Retrieved from https://www.ncsbn.org/Proceedings_from_ Nursing_College_Symposium.pdf

Ragged Edge Online. (1999). The disabilities act covers all of us. Retrieved from http:// www.raggededgemagazine.com/extra/edgextraburgdorf.htm

Reinhart, R. J. (2020). Nurses continue to rank highest in honesty, ethics. *Gallup*. Retrieved from https://news.gallup.com/poll/274673/nurses-continue-rate-highest-honesty-ethics.aspx

Rush University. (n.d.). Disability rights and accessibility programs. Retrieved from https://www.rushu.rush.edu/equal-opportunity-disability-rights-and-accessibility/disability-rights-and-accessibility-programs

Saha, S., Arbelaez, J. J., & Cooper, L. A. (2003). Patient–physician relationships and racial disparities in the quality of health care. *American Journal of Public Health, 93*(10), 1,713–1,719. doi:10.2105/ajph.93.10.1713

Saha, S., Komaromy, M., Koepsell, T. D., & Bindman, A. B. (1999). Patient-physician racial concordance and the perceived quality and use of health care. *Archives of Internal Medicine, 159*(9), 997–1,004.

Saha, S., Taggart, S. H., Komaromy, M., & Bindman, A. B. (2000). Do patients choose physicians of their own race? *Health Affairs, 19*(4), 76–83. doi:10.1377/hlthaff.19.4.76

Schnittker, J., & Liang, K. (2006). The promise and limits of racial/ethnic concordance in physician-patient interaction. *Journal of Health Politics, Policy & Law, 31*(4), 811–838. doi:10.1215/03616878-2006-004

Shapiro, J. P. (1993). *No pity: People with disabilities forging a new civil rights movement*. New York, NY: Crown.

Smith, M. (2009). *Technical standards and essential functions*. Chicago, IL: National Organization of Nurses with Disabilities.

Stein, M. A. (2004). Same struggle, different difference: ADA accommodations as antidiscrimination. *University of Pennsylvania Law Review, 153*(2), 579–673. doi: 10.2307/4150664

Steinmetz, E. (2006). Americans with disabilities: 2002 household economic studies. *United States Census Bureau*. Retrieved from https://www.census.gov/prod/2006pubs/p70-107.pdf

Stolzenberg, E. B., Eagan, K., Romo, E., Tamargo, E. J., Aragon, M. C., Luedke, M., & Kang, N. (2019). The American freshman: National norms fall 2018. *University of California Los Angeles (UCLA) Higher Education Research Institute (HERI)*. Retrieved from https://heri.ucla.edu/monographs/TheAmericanFreshman2018.pdf

Street, R. L., O'Malley, K. J., Cooper, L. A., & Haidet, P. (2008). Understanding concordance in patient-physician relationships: Personal and ethnic dimensions of shared identity. *Annals of Family Medicine, 6*(3), 198–205. doi:10.1370/afm.821

Thierer, T., & Meyerowitz, C. (2005). Education of dentists in the treatment of patients with special needs. *Journal of the California Dental Association, 33*(9), 723–729.

Union of the Physically Impaired Against Segregation and the Disability Alliance. (1975). Fundamental principles of disability. Retrieved from https://disability-studies.leeds.ac.uk/wp-content/uploads/sites/40/library/UPIAS-fundamental-principles.pdf

United Nations Department of Economic and Social Affairs. (n.d.). Factsheet on persons with disabilities. Retrieved from https://www.un.org/development/desa/disabilities/resources/factsheet-on-persons-with-disabilities.html

United States Census Bureau. (2012). Nearly 1 in 5 people have a disability in the U.S., Census Bureau Reports. Retrieved from https://www.census.gov/newsroom/releases/archives/miscellaneous/cb12-134.html

US Bureau of Labor Statistics. (2017). Employment projections 2016–2026. Retrieved from https://www.bls.gov/news.release/archives/ecopro_10242017.pdf

US Department of Education Office of Civil Rights. (2011). Students with disabilities preparing for postsecondary education: Know your rights and responsibilities. Retrieved from https://www2.ed.gov/about/offices/list/ocr/transition.html#reproduction

US Department of Labor Office of Disability Employment Policy. (2014). Health care professionals with disabilities career trends, best practices and call-to-action policy roundtable. Retrieved from https://www.dol.gov/sites/dolgov/files/odep/alliances/nondalliancroundtablereport.pdf

US Department of Labor Office of Disability Employment Policy. (2020). Universal Design. Retrieved from https://www.dol.gov/agencies/odep/topics/universal-design

Wakefield, M. (2013). Nurses and the Affordable Care Act: A call to lead. *Sigma*. Retrieved from https://nursingcentered.sigmanursing.org/features/top-stories/Vol39_3_nurses-and-the-affordable-care-act-a-call-to-lead

Waliany, S. (2016). Health professionals with disabilities: Motivating inclusiveness and representation. *AMA Journal of Ethics, 18*(10), 971–974. doi:10.1001/journalofethics.2016.18.10.fred1-1610

World Health Organization. (2011). World report on disability. Retrieved from https://www.who.int/publications/i/item/world-report-on-disability

Yocom, C. (1996). *Validation study: Functional abilities essential for nursing practices.* Chicago, IL: National Council of State Boards of Nursing.

INDEX

NOTE: Page references noted with a *t* are tables.

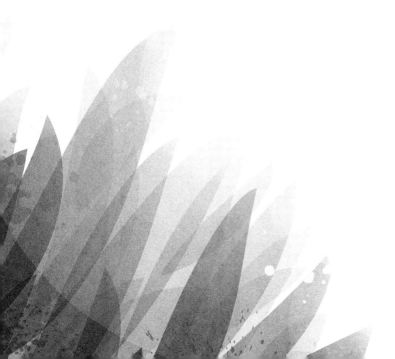

A

J–K

L

M

T

U